APHASIOLOGY

Volume 25 Number 11 November 2011

Special Issue: Discourse in Aphasia
Guest Editor: Heather Harris Wright

CONTENTS

APHASIOLOGY

First published 2011 by Psychology Press

2 Park Square, Milton Park, Abingdon, Oxfordshire OX14 4RN
52 Vanderbilt Avenue, New York, NY 10017

Routledge is an imprint of the Taylor & Francis Group, an informa business

First issued in paperback 2019

ISBN 13: 978-1-138-40391-8 (hbk)
ISBN 13: 978-1-848-72754-0 (pbk)
ISSN 1464-5041.

Typeset by Integra Software Services Pvt. Ltd, India

APHASIOLOGY, 2011, 25 (11), 1283–1285

Discourse in aphasia: An introduction to current research and future directions

Heather Harris Wright

Department of Speech and Hearing Science, Arizona State University, Tempe, AZ USA

Discourse has been defined as any language that is "beyond the boundaries of isolated sentences" (Ulatowska & Olness, 2004, p. 300) and "a set of utterances aimed at conveying a message among interlocutors . . . [it] may be the most elaborative linguistic activity" (Ska, Duong, & Joanette, 2004, p. 302). Discourse production requires more than simply generating a continuous stream of linguistic elements (i.e., phonemes, morphemes, content units, syntax). Successful discourse requires combining units of information in a coherent manner to convey a meaningful message. The study of discourse has spanned many disciplines including linguistics, psychology, gerontology, and communication sciences. Discourse is of particular interest to aphasiologists for numerous reasons: (1) adults with aphasia often have difficulty communicating at the discourse level; (2) analyses of discourse abilities in adults with aphasia are an objective method for evaluating how well the individual can communicate with others; and (3) changes in discourse production can be used to evaluate meaningful change in response to treatment. Discourse abilities in aphasia have garnered more attention in recent years. Researchers have applied methods to evaluate discourse in adults with aphasia to better characterise their communication impairments (e.g., for review see Armstrong, 2000; Olness, Metteson, & Stewart, 2010; Stark, 2010; Ulatowska, Reyes, & Santos, 2010). Researchers have also investigated different methods for quantifying meaningful change in communication abilities of adults with aphasia that are often not detectable by standardised aphasia test batteries (e.g., Fox, Armstrong, & Boles, 2009; Goral & Kempler, 2009; Peach & Reuter, 2010). The purpose of this special issue of *Aphasiology* is to highlight current research in discourse in aphasia. The goal is also to challenge researchers to explore structural and functional theoretical perspectives to more comprehensively characterise communication abilities of adults with aphasia, which may subsequently prove to be sensitive to detecting meaningful change as treatment outcomes measures.

To begin this special issue on Discourse in Aphasia, Brian MacWhinney and colleagues present an overview of AphasiaBank, a computerised database that researchers can access to investigate language use of individuals with aphasia. They present an overview of AphasiaBank including the standard elicitation protocol used

Address correspondence to: Heather Harris Wright, Arizona State University, Department of Speech and Hearing Science, P.O. Box 870102, Tempe, AZ 85287-0102, USA. E-mail: heather.wright.1@asu.edu

http://dx.doi.org/10.1080/02687038.2011.613452

and methods employed for transcription and coding. To illustrate different automatic methods for analysing discourse, they report results of sample analyses applied to Cinderella stories produced by individuals with aphasia.

The next set of papers address treatment at the discourse level in adults with aphasia. Mary Boyle reviews the treatment literature and identifies seven empirical investigations that applied treatment at the discourse level to improve word retrieval ability in individuals with aphasia. Generally, across the treatment studies reviewed, word retrieval ability improved for the study participants following treatment; however, the improvement did not always occur for the treated lexical items. Rather, improvements in general processes of word retrieval were found. Further, review of the studies found that discourse treatment approaches improve informativeness of the discourse produced. Daniel Kempler and Mira Goral apply two treatment approaches, drill-based and discourse-based, to two individuals with nonfluent aphasia to evaluate the efficacy of the different treatments for improving word, sentence, and narrative production. Both treatments focused on verb production. Similar to Goral and Kempler's (2009) findings, positive outcomes on measures were found following the discourse-based treatment. The two study participants improved on word level (number of verbs, verb diversity), sentence level (number of complete utterances, number of grammatical utterances), and discourse level (global coherence, local coherence) measures following the discourse-based treatment but not the drill-based treatment.

The next several papers focus on quantifying discourse production in aphasia by considering different discourse elicitation tasks and different methods for analysing discourse. Elizabeth Armstrong and colleagues apply detailed semantic and syntactic analyses to monologic and dialogic discourse samples collected from two individuals with aphasia. They report finding greater productivity and complexity in monologues compared to dialogues. Andrea Marini and colleagues demonstrate the advantages and usefulness of a multilevel procedure, grounded in linguistic and psychological theories, for documenting change over time in two individuals with aphasia that is not captured by standardised aphasia tests. Gloria Streit Olness and Hanna Ulatowska provide a partial framework for guiding discourse research. They suggest considering qualitative frameworks with quantitative approaches to develop reliable and valid methods for evaluating discourse. They demonstrate this by discussing how personal stories are useful for evaluating coherence in individuals with aphasia. Finally, Gerasimos Fergadiotis and Heather Harris Wright apply a computational method for quantifying lexical diversity in discourse samples collected from adults with and without aphasia. They found that lexical diversity in individuals with aphasia is influenced by the type of discourse elicitation task used.

We end this special issue of *Aphasiology* with Davida Fromm and colleagues' manuscript. They describe evaluative responses by individuals with chronic aphasia about their speech, and they discuss their findings within social models of aphasia therapy. They found that individuals with aphasia had a larger percent of positive responses than negative responses about their speech. They also report that aphasia severity was significantly associated with type of response; those with less severe aphasia had more positive responses.

The work presented in this special issue represents a sampling of the current research in discourse in aphasia. Armstrong and colleagues suggest that their findings raise more questions than answers; this may be true and applicable to the results reported by the authors of the other manuscripts included in this issue. As such, the current research provides a guide for future investigations. As researchers continue to characterise the communication impairments of adults with aphasia, they need to consider their findings within theoretical frameworks.

In future investigations it is clinically important for researchers to establish reliable and valid methods for analysing discourse in aphasia. As demonstrated by Fergadiotis and Wright, and also Armstrong and colleagues, the discourse elicitation task used needs to be considered as well, since many linguistic processes (e.g., vocabulary diversity) are sensitive to task type. We also need to continue establishing reliable and valid clinician-friendly methods; such as on-line transcription-less approaches and computational linguistic approaches. Finally, further investigations of theoretically driven, discourse-based treatments that invoke meaningful change in communication abilities of adults with aphasia are warranted; as are treatment outcome measures to quantify the meaningful changes.

REFERENCES

Armstrong, E. (2000). Aphasic discourse analysis: The story so far. *Aphasiology*, *14*(9), 875–892. doi: 10.1080/02687030050127685

Fox, S., Armstrong, E., & Boles, L. (2009). Conversational treatment in mild aphasia: A case study. *Aphasiology*, *23*, 951–964. doi: 10.1080/02687030802669526

Goral, M., & Kempler, D. (2009). Training verb production in communicative context: Evidence from a person with chronic non-fluent aphasia. *Aphasiology*, *23*, 1383–1397. doi: 10.1080/02687030802235203

Olness, G. S., Metteson, S. E., & Stewart, C. T. (2010). "Let me tell you the point": How speakers with aphasia assign prominence to information in narratives. *Aphasiology*, *24*, 697–708. doi: 10.1080/02687030903438524

Peach, R. K., & Reuter, K. A. (2010). A discourse-based approach to semantic feature analysis for the treatment of aphasic word retrieval failures. *Aphasiology*, *24*, 971–990. doi: 10.1080/02687030903058629

Ska, B., Duong, A., & Joanette, Y. (2004). Discourse impairments. In R. D. Kent (Ed.), *The MIT encyclopedia of communication disorders* (pp. 302–304), Cambridge, MA: The MIT Press.

Stark, J. A. (2010). Content analysis of the fairy tale Cinderella – A longitudinal single case study of narrative production: "From rags to riches". *Aphasiology*, *24*, 709–724. doi: 10.1080/02687030903524729

Ulatowska, H. K., & Olness, G. S. (2004). Discourse. In R. D. Kent (Ed.), *The MIT encyclopedia of communication disorders* (pp. 300–302), Cambridge, MA: The MIT Press.

Ulatowska, H. K., Reyes, B. A., & Santos, T. O. (2010). Stroke narratives in aphasia: The role of reported speech. *Aphasiology*, *25*, 93–105. doi: 10.1080/02687031003714418

APHASIOLOGY, 2011, 25 (11), 1286–1307

AphasiaBank: Methods for studying discourse

Brian MacWhinney[1], Davida Fromm[1], Margaret Forbes[1], and Audrey Holland[2]

[1]Department of Psychology, Carnegie Mellon University, Pittsbrugh, PA, USA
[2]Department of Speech, Language, and Hearing Sciences, University of Arizona, Tucson, AZ, USA

Background: AphasiaBank is a computerised database of interviews between persons with aphasia (PWAs) and clinicians. By February 2011 the database had grown to include 145 PWAs and 126 controls from 12 sites across the United States. The data and related analysis programs are available free over the web.
Aims: The overall goal of AphasiaBank is the construction of a system for accumulating and sharing data on language usage by PWAs. To achieve this goal we have developed a standard elicitation protocol, and systematic automatic and manual methods for transcription, coding, and analysis.
Methods & Procedures: We present sample analyses of transcripts from the retelling of the Cinderella story. These analyses illustrate the application of our methods for the study of phonological, lexical, semantic, morphological, syntactic, temporal, prosodic, gestural, and discourse features.
Outcomes & Results: AphasiaBank will allow researchers access to a large, shared database that can facilitate hypothesis testing and increase methodological replicability, precision, and transparency.
Conclusions: AphasiaBank will provide researchers with an important new tool in the study of aphasia.

Keywords: Aphasia classification; Transcript analysis; Corpus analysis; Elicitation protocols; Gesture analysis; Databases.

AphasiaBank is a computerised database of interviews between aphasic participants and clinicians. These interviews are collected using a consistent protocol format. The video recordings are then transcribed in the CHAT format (MacWhinney, 2000) and each utterance is linked to the corresponding segment in the video recordings. These linked transcripts are made available to AphasiaBank members for further analysis and playback over the web. The collection of AphasiaBank materials began in 2007. By February 2011 we had protocols from 145 persons with aphasia (PWAs),[1]

[1]Our thanks to Dan Kempler (Emerson College), Cynthia Thompson (Northwestern University), and Susan Jackson (University of Kansas) for contributing AphasiaBank protocols from their participants. We also thank Heather Wright (Arizona State University), Darlene Williamson (Stroke Comeback

Address correspondence to: Brian MacWhinney, Carnegie Mellon University, Department of Psychology, 5000 Forbes Avenue, Pittsburgh, PA 15213, USA. E-mail: macw@cmu.edu
This project is funded by NIH_NIDCD grant R01-DC008524 (2007-2012).

http://dx.doi.org/10.1080/02687038.2011.589893

as well as 126 control or comparison participants.[2] The access to transcripts and video materials is password-restricted to AphasiaBank members, but membership is automatically granted to all researchers studying aphasia on request. Access to the programs, manuals, and other resources is open and free to everyone.

In this article we explain how to use the CLAN (Computerised Language Analysis) programs (MacWhinney, 2000) to analyse phonological, lexical, phonological, morphosyntactic, discourse, and gestural patterns in the database. Several publications have already made use of the AphasiaBank database and CLAN programs. MacWhinney, Fromm, Holland, Forbes, and Wright (2010) conducted various lexical analyses of the segment of the protocol in which PWAs describe the Cinderella story. Fergadiotis, Wright, and Capilouto (2011) examined lexical diversity in younger versus older participants across different discourse types using CLAN analyses, but not with AphasiaBank data. Fergadiotis and Wright (2011) used similar methods to analyse AphasiaBank protocol data. Finally, Fromm et al. (2011) studied responses of PWAs to queries about their speech. Segments of these publications will be used as illustrations of the types of analyses that can be conducted.

FORMATION OF THE APHASIABANK SYSTEM

AphasiaBank has been designed to replicate and extend the organisational model established by the Child Language Data Exchange System (CHILDES) for the field of child language acquisition. The CHILDES Project, directed by Brian MacWhinney and funded by NIH/NICHD since 1987, is an international cooperative venture involving over 800 active users and 4000 affiliated members located in over 30 countries. Most new empirical studies of child language production rely on the analysis of data from the CHILDES database and the majority of theoretical papers on language that make reference to production data are now based on the use of the CHILDES database. A recent count located over 3500 published articles based on the use of CHILDES data or programs. The system provides users access to a set of programs (CLAN), a database (CHILDES), a transcription system (CHAT), documentation, and an electronic discussion group (chibolts@googlegroups.com) for communicating on issues in language analysis. The form of these tools has been shaped by continual input from active members of the system.

Work on establishing a system of this type for the study of aphasia started in 2005 with a planning meeting of 20 senior aphasia researchers. At this meeting participants specified the shape of the AphasiaBank protocol and outlined methods for data sharing and possible computational analyses. The AphasiaBank grant, prepared by Brian MacWhinney and Audrey Holland, was funded in 2007. Workshops with senior aphasia researchers have continued on a yearly basis to advise on a large number of issues including protocol development, language transcription, error coding, discourse analysis strategies, and future directions. The AphasiaBank website at http://talkbank.org/AphasiaBank/ is the primary source for all AphasiaBank related materials (e.g., transcripts, videos, computer programs, manuals, transcription

Center), Gretchen Szabo (Adler Aphasia Center), Roberta Elman (Aphasia Center of California), Denise McCall (SCALE), and Maura Silverman (TAP) for helping us administer the AphasiaBank protocol to the participants at their respective institutions.

[2]Thanks to Heather Wright, Gilson Capilouto (University of Kentucky), and Dan Kempler for their contributions of protocols for control participants.

training, IRB guidelines, ground rules). In addition an AphasiaBank Google Group (currently with 98 members) is used for purposes of information dissemination and discussion of topics relevant to the project.

THE APHASIABANK PROTOCOL

The central goal of the AphasiaBank project is the creation of a shared database of multimedia interactions for studying communication in aphasia. Because of the diversity of clinical patterns in aphasia we considered it important to implement a standard protocol to achieve maximal comparability across participants. To that end we have developed a tightly specified data collection protocol that is being consistently implemented at all participating AphasiaBank research sites. The protocol consists of four different discourse elicitation tasks: personal narratives, picture descriptions, story telling, and procedural discourse. We chose to focus on narrative and procedural discourse in order to maximise task comparability across participants. In the future we expect to include additional methods for collecting conversational discourse.

A script was developed to keep the prompts consistent across investigators. The script includes a second-level prompt to use if a participant does not respond in 10 seconds. A troubleshooting script is also available for participants who still cannot respond and need additional prompting with simplified questions. To maximise comparability across sessions the investigator makes every effort to be as silent as possible during administration of the protocol, while giving maximal non-verbal encouragement. Participants are given as much time as they need for their responses. The protocol is administered in a single session and the session is recorded on video, using a set of guidelines to maintain high audio and video recording quality. These guidelines, which are posted at the AphasiaBank website, specify details regarding the video equipment to be used, the configuration of the equipment, and methods for creation of computer files from the video output. There are four discourse tasks:

1. Personal narratives. These are elicited by asking the PWAs about their speech, their stroke, their recovery, and an important event in their lives. Control participants are asked about an illness or injury, their recovery from that illness or injury, any experience they have had with people who have trouble communicating, and an important event in their lives.
2. Picture descriptions. Participants are shown three black and white drawings. They are asked to look at the picture and tell a story with a beginning, middle, and end (Wright & Capilouto, 2009). The first picture stimulus is a four-panelled picture of a child playing with a soccer ball and breaking a window, the second is a six-panelled picture of a child refusing an umbrella and getting caught in the rain, and the third is the Nicholas and Brookshire (1993) picture of a cat stuck in a tree. A fourth picture, a colour photo of a flood rescue scene, was used for the first 2 years of the project and then discontinued because many participants were having trouble interpreting the picture.
3. Story telling. Participants are shown a paperback picture book of Cinderella (Grimes, 2005), with the words covered up. They are told to look through the book to remember how the story goes. Then the book is taken away and they are asked to tell as much of the story as they can.
4. Procedural discourse. Participants are asked to describe how they would make a peanut butter and jam [jelly] sandwich. (Test sites outside the United States may

substitute another simple food preparation.) A stimulus picture with photographs of peanut butter, bread, and jam [jelly] is available for use with participants who need extra help.

Although the current samples are all in English, samples are also being collected in Cantonese, Mandarin, German, and Swedish. Inclusion criteria for PWAs have been limited (with few exceptions) to individuals whose aphasia results from a stroke that can be verified through neuroimaging or a clear medical diagnosis. Extensive demographic data (51 fields) have been collected on each participant and are available to AphasiaBank members at the website. A total of 10 of the PWAs had a second administration of the protocol done approximately 1 year following the initial administration.

In addition to the demographic data, three standardised measures are administered to PWAs: (1) the Aphasia Quotient (AQ) subtests from the Western Aphasia Battery-Revised (WAB; Kertész, 2007); (2) the short form of the Boston Naming Test-Second Edition (Kaplan, Goodglass, & Weintraub, 2001); and (3) the Verb Naming Test from the Northwestern Assessment of Verbs and Sentences-Revised (Thompson, 2011). We also administer a non-standardised repetition test, developed to assess word-level and sentence-level repetition skills. All testing, with the exception of the WAB, is recorded on video. The control participants are tested with the Mini-Mental State Exam (Folstein, Folstein, & Fanjiang, 2002) and the Geriatric Depression Scale (Brink et al., 1982) to rule out cognitive impairment and depression. Test results are also available to AphasiaBank members in a master spreadsheet on the AphasiaBank website.

Transcription and coding

Before being included in AphasiaBank the discourse samples from both PWAs and controls go through a detailed process of transcription, coding, and checking. Transcription is done using the CHAT format (MacWhinney, 2000) that has been developed over the last 30 years for use in a variety of disciplines such as first language acquisition, second language acquisition, classroom discourse, and conversation analysis. CHAT is designed to operate closely with the CLAN programs, which are also described in MacWhinney (2000). These programs allow for the analysis of a wide range of linguistic and discourse structures, some of which will be described in this article. The CLAN program, along with updated electronic versions of the CHAT and CLAN manuals, can be downloaded from the AphasiaBank website at http://talkbank.org/AphasiaBank. That site also provides a transcription training manual that was prepared specifically for AphasiaBank purposes.

For detailed transcription we rely on CLAN's Walker Controller function that allows the transcriber to replay segments of the video. This replaying can be done with a variable window and a variable lag. When desired, replay can be controlled through a foot pedal attached to the USB port on the computer. Figure 1 illustrates the set-up for transcription with a transcript window, the QuickTime video/audio window, and the Walker Controller window. The Walker Controller is set here to replay stretches of 4 seconds three times and then move on with a backspace of 1 second. It is also set here to play the media at 80% real speed.

During transcription, utterances are segmented based on criteria derived from syntax, intonation, pauses, and semantics, in accord with the analysis of Berndt, Wayland,

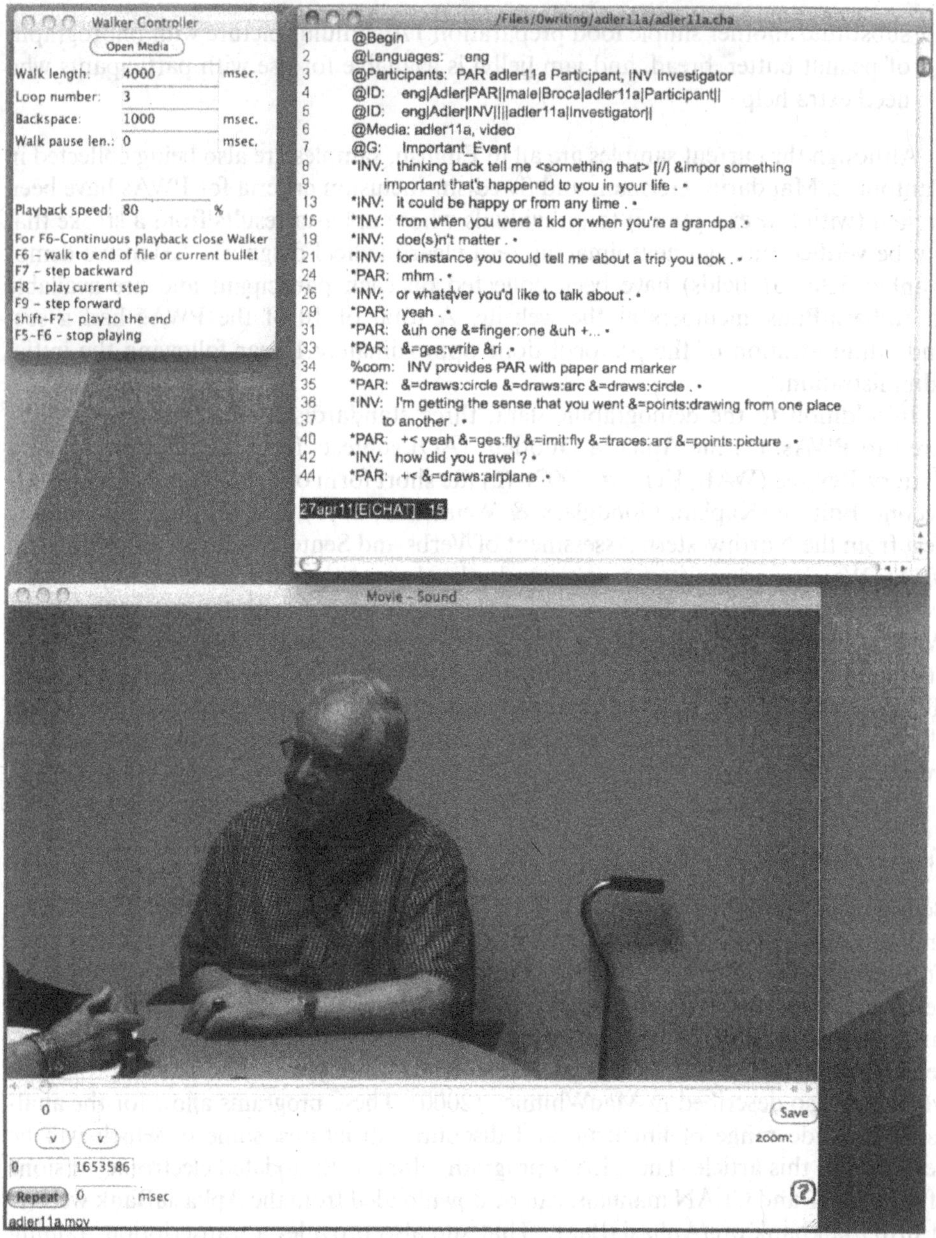

Figure 1. Window arrangement for transcribing using walker controller.

Rochon, Saffran, and Schwartz (2000). The CHAT transcription format includes conventions for marking linguistic behaviours such as word repetitions, revisions, fillers, gestures, sound fragments, and unintelligible output. Transcriptions are further elaborated by detailed coding for error type. This coding is done by certified, licensed speech-language pathologists with clinical and research experience in aphasia. For word-level errors we code errors in six categories: phonology, semantics, neologism, dysfluency, morphology, and formal lexical features (e.g., article errors). Within each category word-level errors are coded further to indicate whether the error was a word or non-word, the target was known or unknown, a suffix was missing, and more. Errors that are not real words are transcribed using IPA. The error code also indicates if the error was repeated or retraced by the speaker within the utterance. The sentence-level codes capture empty speech, circumlocution, jargon, agrammatism and paragrammatism, and perseveration. A complete list of the error codes, definitions, and examples is available at the AphasiaBank website.

Checking

Every transcript goes through four levels of checking. The first level relies on the CHECK program that is built into the CLAN editor. To run this checker the transcriber types escape-L and looks to see if any errors are reported. We run this initial check several times during the production of a transcript. After initial completion transcripts are then reviewed by at least two transcribers for accuracy before being uploaded to the website. For the transcripts from PWAs one of those reviewers is always a certified, licensed speech-language pathologist. The third level of checking relies on part-of-speech tagging through the MOR program, which is described below. If a transcript can be run through MOR without errors we know that the transcript has no unrecognisable words. In effect, MOR serves as a filter for detecting misspellings and other incorrect lexical forms. The fourth level of checking relies on the Chatter program to test for complete adherence to the CHAT XML Schema.

All of the data in AphasiaBank have been run through all four levels of checking. Much of this work has been done at Carnegie Mellon, but we have also been able to train 14 transcribers at various sites to make reliable use of the CHAT coding system for AphasiaBank data. For researchers with training in language analysis and good familiarity with computers it takes about 3 days to learn to transcribe in CHAT for AphasiaBank data.

Morphological tagging

After completing transcription we conduct part-of-speech tagging using the MOR program. Analysis through MOR has two important functions. First, as we noted above, MOR acts as a filter against misspellings and other incorrect lexical forms. Because each word must have some recognisable morphological structure, MOR will catch and list many typos and other errors in transcription, which can then be corrected. Often transcribers wish to note that a word has a deviant phonological shape. At the same time they need to relate that shape to some standard word form. To do this CHAT uses a replacement form structure. For example, a deviant production of the word "pretzel" as "pezzle" can be transcribed orthographically or phonetically: pezzle [: pretzel] or pɛzəl@u [: pretzel]. The MOR program will use the form in the replacement brackets, ignoring the preceding form. Another way of bridging the gap between actual productions and the forms seen by MOR is to enclose omitted material in parentheses, as in *(be)cause* for the word "because". Additionally, transcribers can match speaker's productions more closely to well-formed targets by using marks for repetition and retracing such as [/] and [//]. Faithful use of these and other transcription devices can greatly improve the quality of a transcription and facilitate the accurate running of MOR and POST.

The second function of MOR involves the use of the part-of-speech tags inserted by MOR for other programs. These tags provide a gateway to a wide variety of further automatic analyses of morphology, lexicon, and syntax. For the data currently in AphasiaBank, MOR analysis has been completed. However, it is important for users to understand how this analysis was constructed and how to interpret the tags.

We have developed MOR taggers for English, Spanish, German, French, Italian, Japanese, Cantonese, and Mandarin. For data currently in AphasiaBank we rely on the English MOR program. The results of the MOR tagger are then disambiguated using the POST statistical disambiguator (Parisse & Le Normand, 2000). POST uses the context before and after the word to assign part-of-speech to ambiguous cases. After running MOR, POST, and CHECK (to ensure that the output is complete and technically accurate), the transcript then appears with a new tier, %mor, under each speaker tier, giving the lexical and morphological tags for each word on the main speaker tier. These morphological codes can then be used to automatically compute a variety of indices and other linguistic analyses.

To judge the accuracy of tagging with MOR and POST we reviewed six control transcripts (over 20,000 total words) and did manual morphological tagging on a %trn line. Results demonstrated 98.87% agreement between the part-of-speech tagging done automatically by CLAN and that done manually. However, for new samples we expect accuracy to decline to about 98%, because statistical taggers always do better on training data than on new data. For transcripts from PWAs the level of tagging accuracy depends on the type of aphasia and other characteristics of the individual speaker. For participants with anomia or mild agrammatism, morphological tagging accuracy levels are close to those for controls. For participants with more severe agrammatism it is also possible to achieve high levels of accuracy for part-of-speech tagging, because the syntactic constructions being used are often quite simple, as in child language data where tagging of productions from children between 2 and 3 years of age has an accuracy level of about 96%. For participants with jargon aphasia it is often difficult to map productions onto standard word forms. For this group the tagging of word forms for the traditional part-of-speech categories is, by definition, less reliable. However, using the CHAT error coding system, the neologisms and word approximations of speakers with jargon aphasia can be classified systematically into various non-word categories and the remaining conventional words can be tagged with conventional tags.

The following example shows a few lines from a language sample from a participant describing his stroke, showing speaker lines (INV for investigator and PAR for participant) and their corresponding %mor lines. Some CHAT symbols that appear on the main speaker tier include: [/] for repetition, [//] for revision, &= before gestures or simple events (e.g., &=laughs, &=sighs, &=sneezes), and & before sound fragments and fillers. On the %mor line, the part of speech (e.g., aux for auxiliary, pro for pronoun, v for verb) comes before the vertical bar and the word used by the speaker from the main tier. Suffixes are attached to the word (e.g., -PROG for progressive, -PAST for regular past).

```
*INV:  can you tell me what you remember about it ?
%mor:  aux|can pro|you v|tell pro|me pro:wh|what pro|you v|remember prep|about
       pro|it ?
*PAR:  I remember falling off the chair and [/] and &w &w &wonder &won
       wondering what happened to me.
%mor:  pro|I v|remember n:gerund|fall-GERUND prep|off det|the n|chair conj:coo|and
       n:gerund|wonder-GERUND pro:wh|what v|happen-PAST prep|to pro|me.
```

*PAR: and I couldn't get up &=laughs.
%mor: conj:coo|and pro|I aux|could~neg|not v|get adv:loc|up.
*PAR: and I [//] it was morning.
%mor: conj:coo|and pro|it v:cop|be&PAST&13S n|morning.
*PAR: and &uh &um it wasn't until the afternoon that I called Alice.
%mor: conj:coo|and pro|it v:cop|be&PAST&13S~neg|not prep|until det|the n|afternoon rel|that pro|I v|call-PAST n:prop|Alice.
*PAR: but I couldn't say anything.
%mor: conj: coo|but pro|I aux|could~neg|not v|say pro:indef|anything.

Transcripts that have been tagged using MOR and POST can then be further analysed for syntactic structure using the GRASP Program (Sagae, Davis, Lavie, MacWhinney, & Wintner, 2010). This program takes the words on the %mor line and relates them in terms of a set of 34 binary syntactic dependency relations such as SUBJect, ADJunct, MODifier, and so on. The extraction of these relations allows researchers to study the use of syntactic patterns in aphasia and also supports the automatic computation of morphosyntactic profiles such as DSS (Lee, 1966) and IPSyn (Sagae, Lavie, & MacWhinney, 2005; Scarborough, 1990).

ILLUSTRATIVE ANALYSES

In this section we present a series of analyses of segments of the Cinderella story, designed to illustrate how we can analyse AphasiaBank transcripts. Our basic goal here is to illustrate the operation of the programs. At the same time, these analyses provide evidence regarding substantive issues in the study of aphasia. CLAN provides 15 analysis programs, each with a wide variety of functions and options. String-search programs can compute frequency counts, key-word and line profiles, mean length of utterance, mean length of turn, type-token ratios, maximum word length counts, maximum utterance length histograms, vocabulary diversity, temporal durations, and so on. The CHAT transcript files include header lines with several fields for demographic information, thereby making it possible to analyse subsets of the entire database based on, for example, sex or aphasia type.

MacWhinney et al. (2010) conducted a number of analyses of AphasiaBank data that focused on the segment of the protocol in which the participant retells the Cinderella story. Those analyses were done using the smaller database ($n = 24$ PWAs, $n = 25$ controls) that was available earlier in the project. Here we extend those analyses to the larger database currently available. The samples used for these analyses include all PWAs who meet these criteria: (1) aphasia caused by stroke; (2) relatively complete demographic and testing data; (3) native speakers of English; and (4) produced at least one utterance in response to the task. At the time of preparation of this manuscript, 90 PWAs met these criteria. We also selected 90 controls who met these criteria: (1) complete demographic data; (2) native speakers of American English; and (3) minimum age of 36.0 years. The characteristics of the PWAs and the controls appear in Table 1. Statistical tests revealed no significant difference between the two groups on the basis of age or education, but a chi-square test resulted in a significant difference, $\chi^2(1) = 5.714$, $p < .05$, between the groups on sex, with a higher ratio of males to females in the PWAs.

Before conducting the lexical frequency analyses, the Cinderella story segments of the transcripts were extracted using the GEM command. This command requires that segments of the transcript be demarcated with @G lines indicating the beginning of an

TABLE 1
Demographic and test data for AphasiaBank participants

	PWA, n=90	*Control, n=90*
Age	64.5 years (*SD*=12.3) range=36–90.7	64.7 years (*SD*=13.8) range=36–87.8
Sex	34 females 56 males	50 females 40 males
Handedness	77 right 7 left 4 ambidextrous 2 unknown	80 right 8 left 2 ambidextrous
Education	15.7 years (*SD*=2.9) range=12–25	15.1 years (*SD*=2.4) range=10–22
Time post-onset	6.6 years (*SD*=6.0) range=0.5–39.2	
Type of aphasia (from Western Aphasia Battery – WAB)	32 anomic 20 Broca 16 conduction 9 Wernicke 8 not aphasic 3 transcortical motor 1 global 1 unavailable	
WAB AQ (aphasia quotient)	71.8 (*SD*=18.9) range=17–97.6	

activity. In this case, @G: Cinderella Story is used to mark the beginning of the participant's retell. In addition, it is necessary to exclude extraneous comments made during the task, such as "wait a second", "can't say it right", and "I know". Those utterances are marked with a sentence level code [+ exc] during transcription. We typed the following command into the CLAN command window to extract the Cinderella retell portion of the transcript.

```
gem +sCinderella +sStory -s"[+ exc]" +g +n +d1 +t*PAR +t%mor +f +re *.cha
```

This command has 11 segments:

gem	calls up the GEM command
+sCinderella +sStory	searches for the words Cinderella and Story
-s"[+ exc]"	excludes utterances coded for exclusion
+ g	selects the @G or @BG segment that has all and only the words specified by the +s option
+n	ends the segment at the next @G in the transcript
+d1	creates output in legal CHAT format
+t*PAR	includes the participant speaker tier
+t%mor	includes the %mor tier
+f	sends output to a new file (with .gem.cex extension)
+re	runs program subdirectories within a folder
*.cha	runs the command on all the .cha files

TABLE 2
Lexical frequency analysis results: Mean, standard deviation, range

		PWA			*Control*		
		All	*Female*	*Male*	*All*	*Female*	*Male*
N		90	34	56	90	50	40
Total words	mean	195.3	223.0	172.9	476.3	490.7	458.3
	SD	157.8	173.8	144.3	291.3	273.3	315.0
	range	1–770	23–770	1–580	33–1659	60–1304	33–1659
Total different words	mean	76.7	88.3	69.6	180.6	183.7	176.8
	SD	47.0	48.0	45.3	81.0	80.6	82.5
	range	1–189	17–186	1–189	25–412	38–412	25–388
VOCD (word stems)	mean	34.5	38.5	31.8	56.7	54.9	59.9
	SD	16.5	15.6	16.2	13.2	11.6	15.1
	range	7.8–65.8	11.8–65.8	7.8–59.2	32.7–92.2	34.6–92.1	32.7–87.8

Lexical frequency analysis

Once we had extracted the relevant segments of the transcript using GEM, we could then proceed with further analyses. Our first set of analyses uses the FREQ program to compute these four forms of lexical frequency analysis: (1) overall sex and group differences, (2) top 10 item differences, (3) noun usage, and (4) verb usage.

Sex and group difference analysis. The first FREQ analysis examined the relative distribution of word forms across participant group and sex. To get the total number of words (tokens) and the number of different words (type), excluding repetitions, revisions, and unintelligible words, the following FREQ command was used.

```
freq +t*PAR -r6 +re +d3 -sxx *.gem.cex
```

The five new components of this command are:

freq	calls up the FREQ command
-r6	excludes repetitions and revisions
+d3	outputs type/token information for analysis in Excel
-sxx	excludes unintelligible words
*.gem.cex	runs the command on all files with the .gem.cex extension

This command can be modified to look specifically at only females (or males) by adding one more element: +t@id="*|female|*" (or +t@id="*|male|*").

Results of the type and token analysis for both PWAs and controls appear in Table 2. One can see that the controls produced more than twice as many total words and different words as the PWAs, $t(178)$, $p < .001$, one-tailed. While one might imagine that females might produce more output than males in their Cinderella story retells, we found no evidence to suggest that was the case. Differences between males and females were not significant in the controls for total number of words, $t(88)$, $p = .69$, or total number of different words, $t(88)$, $p = .60$. Differences between males and females were more pronounced in the PWAs, although they did not reach statistical significance for total number of words, $t(88)$, $p = .08$, or total number of different words, $t(88)$, $p = .06$.

TABLE 3
CLAN output for word frequency: Top 25 words in descending order

PWA – All	*Control – All*	*PWA – Nouns*	*Control – Nouns*	*PWA – Verbs*	*Control – Verbs*
1688 and	3212 the	320 Cinderella	719 Cinderella	663 v:cop|be	1182 v:cop|be
1271 the	3144 and	132 ball	421 prince	291 aux|be	634 aux|be
959 be	1861 be	131 girl	409 ball	204 v|go	530 v|go
637 she	1717 to	126 prince	348 slipper	186 v|have	425 v|have
534 to	1536 she	106 slipper	275 mother	157 v|say	385 v|get
377 a	1148 her	97 mother	268 sister	151 v|get	248 v|say
320 Cinderella	962 a	91 shoe	208 glass	112 aux|do	217 aux|do
316 they	740 go	89 sister	188 dress	95 part|go	217 aux|will
300 go	719 Cinderella	65 dress	164 godmother	93 v|do	199 part|go
296 it	648 they	64 daughter	163 fairy	73 v|want	185 v|come
281 her	614 have	61 woman	160 daughter	64 v|come	154 aux|have
247 then	599 so	58 man	155 home	62 v|find	151 v|find
238 so	581 of	52 home	140 girl	57 v|know	151 v|make
232 have	575 that	48 horse	136 house	56 v|see	142 v|try
217 do	474 in	47 thing	119 time	51 aux|will	127 v|do
205 not	455 it	45 house	118 midnight	49 aux|can	118 v|live
201 but	437 get	44 person	115 pumpkin	39 v|fit	118 v|want
192 I	433 he	42 o'clock	114 mouse	38 aux|have	106 v|see
189 that	421 prince	41 fairy	109 shoe	36 v|take	105 v|fit
169 he	413 ball	40 time	108 woman	34 v|think	103 v|turn
168 say	410 not	39 godmother	103 carriage	33 aux|could	101 aux|can
164 get	374 do	32 sudden	91 foot	32 v|look	97 aux|could
147 of	358 all	31 glass	80 father	30 part|dance	94 v|take
137 ball	348 slipper	30 mouse	76 horse	30 v|dance	90 v|marry
134 oh	319 with	30 pumpkin	71 castle	28 v|make	88 v|know

Top 10 analysis. The second FREQ analysis examined the overlap between groups in terms of the top 10 words used in describing the Cinderella story. MacWhinney et al. (2010) used FREQ to conduct a detailed comparison of the top 10 words in the PWA samples with the top 10 in the control samples. Based on the sample at that time of 24 PWAs and 25 controls, they showed a nearly complete overlap between these lists for the top 10 words, although PWAs had a markedly reduced lexical diversity. Here we extend this analysis to our larger sample of 90 PWAs and 90 controls. The first analysis computes the frequencies of word form occurrences on the %mor line, excluding neologisms and unintelligible words. In cases where PWAs made an error, but the intended word was known (e.g., phonological errors in the pronunciation of "Cinderella", semantic errors such as "foot" for "shoe"), the intended word was used for this analysis. The command we used to construct the overall frequency profile was:

```
freq +t%mor +t*PAR –t* +s@r-*,o-% +u -s@"|-neo,|-unk" +o +f +re *.gem.cex
```

From the output produced by this command we extracted the occurrences of the 25 most-frequent words. The first two columns of Table 3 provide these 25 most-frequent words across all parts of speech for the PWA and control groups' stories.

The previous article reported the top 15 words for the PWAs only. The current larger sample yielded nearly the same list in roughly the same order. Three words—

then, have, and *so*—appeared in the top 15 for this larger group, displacing three—*not, he,* and *I*—from the previous list. In the current analysis the top 25 words are similar for the PWAs and controls with the exception of 5 words: *then, but, I, say,* and *oh* appear in the aphasia list; *in, prince, all, slipper,* and *with* appear in the list for the control participants. Overall, this analysis replicates the results of MacWhinney et al. (2010).

Noun usage. We also examined the frequencies of nouns across the PWA and control groups. To do this, we used the following command to tabulate the frequencies of all nouns, including proper nouns, compound nouns, and nouns with prefixes, collapsing across stems:

```
freq +t%mor +t*PAR –t* +o +s@r-*,|-n:*,|-n,o-% +u +re *.gem.cex
```

The results of this analysis are given in Columns 3 and 4 of Table 3. PWAs produced about half as many (383 vs 661) different nouns as did the controls with about a third the number (3062 vs 8289) of noun tokens (total noun stems). The two lists of most frequently occurring nouns have 20/25 words in common (slightly higher than the 6/10 reported in the previous study). Again, the stories from the PWAs included the words *man, thing, person, o'clock,* and *sudden,* which are not as tightly and specifically linked to the Cinderella story as are the words *midnight, carriage, foot, father,* and *castle* that appear in the controls' top 25. Additionally, in the PWA samples, *girl*, another less-specific word, is the 3rd most frequently occurring noun, as opposed to being 13th in the non-aphasic samples. And the word *glass,* which is used to describe a detailed aspect of the slipper in the Cinderella story, was 23rd on the list of word frequency for the PWAs but 7th on the controls' list. Interestingly, although the PWAs used the word *o'clock* only 41 times, they used *twelve*, in the combination *twelve o'clock,* 35 out of these 41 times. They used the word *twelve* 52 times in all (17 times without the word *o'clock* immediately following) and they used the word *midnight* 19 times. The controls said *midnight* 126 times, *twelve o'clock* together as a unit only 18 times, *twelve* 53 times, and *o'clock* 19 times.

Verb usage. As was the case for nouns, PWAs produced just over half as many (317 vs 590) different verbs as did the controls with just over a third as many total verbs stems in the sample (3657 vs 9371). We used the following command to find all verbs, auxiliaries, and participles, again collapsed across stems:

```
freq +t%mor +t*PAR –t* +o +s"@r-*,|-v*,o-%" +s"@r-*,|-aux,|-aux:*,o%" +s"@r-*,|-
part*,o-%"+u +re *.gem.cex
```

Because it can be difficult for users to remember how to construct complex commands of this type, we have provided a user interface for the construction of the +t and +s switches, as illustrated in Figure 2. The top 25 most frequently occurring verbs in both groups appear in columns 5 and 6 of Table 3. In this case the part of speech label is included to indicate the exact form of the verb (e.g., verb, copula, verb participle, auxiliary). The most frequently occurring verbs have 21/25 words in common across the two groups (higher than the 7/10 reported in the previous study). The stories from the PWAs included more frequent use of the verbs *think, dance* (in verb and participle forms), and *look,* whereas the stories from the controls included more frequent use of the verbs *turn, live, try,* and *marry.*

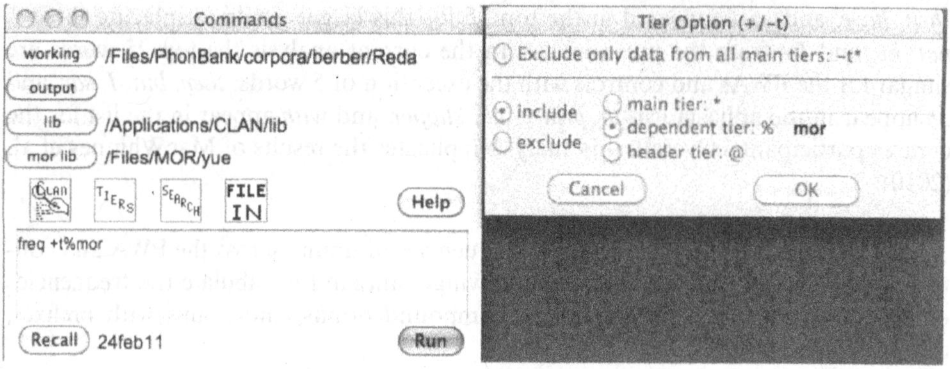

Figure 2. Building the +t switch in the CLAN commands window.

Lexical diversity analysis

One possible consequence of aphasia is a reduction in lexical diversity (Wright, Silverman, & Newhoff, 2003). For example, we may be interested in understanding whether individuals with non-fluent aphasia have a greater reduction in lexical diversity than do individuals with fluent aphasia. Traditionally this feature of aphasic speech has been measured using the type-token ratio (TTR) measure (Holmes & Singh, 1996). However, a major problem with TTR is the fact that it is overly sensitive to sample size, because frequent words only demonstrate their impact in larger samples. Particularly for short samples from individuals with non-fluent aphasia, TTR could provide an inflated estimation of lexical diversity. To address this problem, Malvern, Richards, Chipere, and Purán (2004) developed the VOCD (VOCabulary Diversity) statistic. VOCD corrects the problem with TTR by selecting up to 20 alternative sample sizes for computation of the type ratio. This then allows the program to plot and compare the lexical diversity function independently of some particular sample size. Because VOCD is superior to TTR in this regard, Table 2 reports VOCD scores, rather than TTR scores. One can compute VOCD either from the main speaker line or the %mor line in the CHAT transcript. The advantage of calculating VOCD from the %mor line is that one can do an analysis that focuses on lemmas, rather than word forms. That is, we can treat variant inflected forms of the same base (e.g., *play, playing, played* or *unhappy, happy, happily*) as the same lexical item, thereby obtaining a more accurate measure of lexical diversity. The following command was used to do this analysis, excluding neologisms and unintelligible words as well.

```
vocd +t%mor +t*PAR –t* +s"*|*-%%" +s"*|-&%%" -s@"|-neo,|-unk" +d3 +re *.gem.cex
```

Results of the VOCD analysis also appear in Table 2. VOCD could not be computed in 11 PWA samples and one control sample, because there were not enough tokens for random sampling without replacement. VOCD differences between males and females were not significant for either group but the VOCD difference between groups was significant, $t(178)$. $p < .001$, with PWA samples including about 60% of the lexical diversity seen in the control samples.

Morphosyntactic analysis

Researchers have proposed several systems for analysing control of morphosyntactic markings and patterns in normal and disordered speech. Among the most well-known systems are LARSP (Fletcher & Garman, 1988), DSS (Lee, 1966), IPSyn (Scarborough, 1990), and QPA (Rochon, Saffran, Berndt, & Schwartz, 2000). Because each of these systems requires careful hand analysis, tagging, and coding, they have only been used sparingly in research studies and clinical practice. CLAN's MORtable program provides automatic computation of many of the indices that figure prominently in these earlier hand-coded systems.

The MORtable command works automatically on the %mor line to construct a table of the parts-of-speech that can be opened directly in Excel. The command has this form:

```
mortable +t*PAR +u +re *gem.cex
```

The results appear in Table 4. Looking at the right-hand column with proportions, one can see that the PWA samples were disproportionately low in these parts of speech: reflexive pronouns, possessive pronouns, prepositions, modals, and infinitives. For the bound morphemes that mark regular inflectional morphology (MacWhinney, 1978; Pinker, 1979), the PWA samples were disproportionately low in the use of the superlative, possessive, regular third person singular, and regular past tense.

The output of MORtable can serve as the input to automatic computation of indices such as LARSP, DSS, IPSyn, and QPA. Currently, CLAN provides this type of automatic computation for DSS and IPSyn.

Apart from the across-the-board analyses provided by MORtable, researchers can also conduct targeted analyses of morphosyntactic structures using the COMBO program. COMBO is designed to search for syntactic and collocational patterns with variables across either the main line or the %mor line. In the Cinderella story material extracted by GEM, we searched the groups for the use of these collocations: *once upon a time, happily ever after, glass slipper(s),* and *fairy godmother.* The following COMBO commands were used, using the +r6 option to exclude revisions and repetitions within utterances.

```
combo +t*PAR +re +u +r6 +sonce^upon^a^time *.gem.cex
combo +t*PAR +re +u +r6 +shappily^ever^after *.gem.cex
combo +t*PAR +re +u +r6 +sfairy^godmother *.gem.cex
combo +t*PAR +re +u +r6 +sglass^slipper* *.gem.cex
```

In the PWA samples, *once upon a time* did not occur at all; in the control samples it occurred 13 times. *Happily ever after* occurred only 10 times in the samples from PWAs and 61 times in the control samples. *Glass slipper(s)* occurred together 20 times in the samples from the PWAs and 199 times in the control samples. *Fairy godmother* occurred together 26 times in the PWA samples and 153 times in the control samples. The relative infrequency of these collocations in the PWA samples seems to indicate a diminished use of finer levels of narrative expression. Interestingly, in the PWA samples (excluding revisions and repetitions) the word *fairy* was used 41 times and the word *godmother* appeared 38 times, illustrating that sometimes only one of the words was used and sometimes the words were both produced in the sentence but not as an uninterrupted unit. In the control samples, *fairy* occurred 172 times and *godmother* 169 times, much closer to the 161 times these two words occurred together. Likewise,

TABLE 4
Parts of speech and bound morpheme frequency counts

Parts of speech	*PWA (90)*	*Control (90)*	*PWA/Control*
wh-words	105	236	.44
adjectives	667	1621	.41
adverbs	1244	2770	.45
auxiliaries	442	1022	.43
complements	0	0	–
conjunctions	2155	4243	.50
determiners	1759	4479	.39
infinitives	311	1022	.30
modals	142	472	.30
nouns	3062	8289	.37
negatives	205	410	.50
prepositions	955	3493	.27
pronouns	2370	5062	.47
possessive pronouns	131	628	.21
reflexive pronouns	6	37	.16
quantifier, determiner:number	454	782	.58
verbs, copulas, participles	3073	7877	.39
Bound morphemes	*PWA (90)*	*Control (90)*	*PWA/Control*
3rd person singular – regular	247	1191	.20
3rd person singular – irregular	476	807	.59
past tense – regular	203	743	.27
past tense – irregular	1023	2059	.49
comparative	11	22	.50
superlative	0	13	0
plural – regular	447	1147	.39
plural – irregular	81	215	.37
possessive	17	119	.14
perfect participle – regular	95	261	.36
perfect participle – irregular	47	187	.25
progressive	318	763	.41

the word *glass* occurred 31 times and *slipper(s)* 100 times in the samples from the PWAs; and 217 times and 365 times, respectively in the control samples.

Error analysis

To capture word-level and sentence-level errors we apply an extensive coding system that has been shaped specifically for AphasiaBank transcripts. Using FREQ, one can search for variant forms of production of a word such as *Cinderella* with the command below:

```
freq +t*PAR +s"Cinderella*" +d6 +re +u *.gem.cex
```

Results reveal that the word *Cinderella* (and *Cinderella's*) was produced by the PWAs 349 times (including repetitions and retracings), and 23% (79) of those were not correct. In only six cases was an attempt made to revise the incorrect production within the same sentence. In no cases was the same error repeated within the same sentence. Some of the errors met the strict criteria used in this project for phonological

TABLE 5
Error productions of Cinderella (with frequency if greater than 1)

Phonological (non-word), N = 31				
sɪndəwɛlə (6)	twɪndəɹɛlə	sɪndɚlɛlə	sɛndɚɛlə	
sɝndɚɛlə	sɪndʒəɹɛlə	sɪldəɹɛlə	sɪndəlɛlə	
sɪnəɹɛlə (5)	sɪndəɹɛləz (3)	dɪndəɹɛlə	swɪndəɹɛlə	
kɪndɚɛlə	sɪndəɹɛlədz	sɪndɚɛtlə	sɪntəɹɛlə	
sɪnbɚɛlə	sɪndɚɛldə	tsɪndɚɛlə	ɪndəɹɛlə	
Neologism (known target), N = 41				
səkɝəndɪd	sɪljɚɛndə	sɪndəwɛɾə (2)	sɪndəɹɛnɪlə	sɪndəɹʌndid
sɪbɛlə	sɛlərɛlə	sɪnəwɛlə	sɪləwɛlə	sʌntɚɛɹɪ
dɹɪnθɪ	sɪlədərɛlə	twɪndəwɛlə	sɪləwɪlə	sɪpɚɛɹɪ
sɪndɑɹɪlɛdɚəl	kɑɹɪtəl	swɪnwɛlə	sɪləwɪlɪpəpə	sɪnjɚlɹɛlə
ɛnsɚsɛtɚ	sɪndəwɛdɚ (3)	kɹɛləlɛlə	sɪndəwɪlə	tʃɪndɚɛtlə
sɝndɚdɹɛləl	sɪndəɹɛdɚ	sɛndɚɛlɪ	sɪndəwɛlwɪn	tsɪndɚɛlgə
sɪndəlɛlɚ	dɪwɛdɚ	sɪndɚlə	sɪndəwɛlwə	tsɪndɚɛtlə
		dʒusinə	tsɪndəɹɛlɪ	sɪlə
Semantic related, N = 5				
Cinder (2)	Cindy	Cin (2)		
Semantic unrelated, N = 2				
weather (2)				

errors, but most did not. For an error on a multi-syllabic word to be coded as a phonological error, the error must have complete syllable matches on all but one syllable, and the syllable with the error must match on two out of the three elements of the syllable (onset, vowel nucleus, coda). So, for example, *Cindewella* and *Cinberella* would be considered phonological non-word errors (coded [* p:n]), but *Cillewilla, Cellerella,* and *Swinwella* would be considered neologisms with a known target (coded [* n:k]). (All non-word errors in the transcripts are transcribed in IPA.) A list of all *Cinderella* error productions by error type is given in Table 5.

A variety of interesting error analyses could be conducted, for example, looking at related versus unrelated semantic paraphasias, the number of phonological errors in neologisms for known targets, the number of errors that are repeated, the ways in which errors are revised, errors on particular parts of speech such as pronouns, proportions of errors in free speech versus picture descriptions, and errors by type or severity of aphasia. We will report on a few of these for purposes of illustration. Using the command below, a list of related and unrelated semantic errors was generated.

```
freq +s"[\* s:r*]" +s"[\* s:ur*]" +u +re +t*PAR +d6 *.gem.cex
```

Results revealed 230 semantically related errors and 10 semantically unrelated errors in the Cinderella stories by the PWAs. In 80 cases attempts were made to revise the error within the same utterance, and in 8 cases the error was repeated within the same utterance. Examples of the unrelated semantic errors are: *trucks* for *dress, weather* for *Cinderella, words* for *wand, building* for *carriage,* and *bliss* for *slipper.* The most commonly occurring related semantic errors are *he* for *she, she* for *he, him* for *her, his* for *her, foot* for *shoe, mother* for *stepmother,* and *princess* for *prince.*

The preponderance of pronoun for pronoun substitutions can be investigated further using the command below to generate a list of pronouns and errors.

```
freq +t%mor +t*PAR -t* +d6 +o +s"@r-*,|-*pro,o-%" +s"@r-*,|-*pro:*,o-%" +re +u
*.gem.cex
```

Errors occurred on 86 of 2579 pronoun productions (excluding repetitions and revisions) in the aphasia stories. In 72 of those cases (84%) the error was another pronoun; in 1 case the error was *in* for *it*, which could be considered phonological or semantic, but still not another pronoun; 6 errors were purely phonological in nature (e.g., *see* for *she, bay* for *they*); 4 pronouns were produced with unknown targets (referents); 2 were produced dysfluently (with syllable insertions); and 1 error was phonological in nature but was coded as a neologism because it had multiple element changes (*herfers* for *herself*).

Another form of error analysis tracks the ways in which PWAs attempt to produce the collocations most relevant to the story. Earlier, we saw that collocations like *glass slipper, happily ever after,* and *fairy godmother* were relatively rare in the PWA samples. When we look at the productions of these forms, we see that they are often produced as errors. For example, *glass slipper(s)* were called *glass skipper, glass sippers, glass ball,* and *glass crystal. Fairy godmother* appeared as *fairy god, fairy grandmother, fairy govmother, fairy mother, grairy godmother, sairy godmother,* and *firey godmother.* Examples of some paraphasic errors for *happily ever after* appear below.

*PAR: they live hevry [: happily] ever after.
*PAR: &uh and they're &maf hæfɪplɪ@u [: happily] ever after.

While very few PWAs managed to say *happily ever after,* many of them attempted to communicate the concept at the end of their stories in a variety of alternative ways, some of which are shown below.

*PAR: he's very happy with her.
*PAR: and a &h happy life &=laughs.
*PAR: and so &um the prince and &uh Cinderella &i <is no> [//] was &uh very &h happy all [/] all the way through.
*PAR: yes but &uh gɔt@u and Cinderella hɪv@u [: live] happy together.
*PAR: and &um &um the man and the [//] &uh sɪndəwɛdɚ@u [: Cinderella] ɔlweɪ@u [: always] &b happy ever æfə□@u [: after].
*PAR: and then he [//] she is &um &uh in the end had a very in happy &w &uh place.
*PAR: well she wears [: lives] &ev happy of ever.
*PAR: &hap happy [/] happy something yeah.
*PAR: and &uh &a &=fingers:writes æpɪ@u [: happy] [/] æpɪ@u [: happy] &=hand:no no [//] &uh &eh and &eh marriage.
*PAR: &=sighs &hm (.) &uh &=sighs I think &=ges:unsure Cinderella's hævə@u [: happy] ever after.
*PAR: and so she's happy ever after.
*PAR: <and they> [/] &ha [x 3] and they (.) happy ever after.
*PAR: and so the (.) married and [/] &=shrugs and &uh married &h after.

Gesture analysis

There have been a number of analyses of the use of gesture by people with aphasia in spontaneous communicative situations (Glosser, Wiener, & Kaplan, 1986; Goodwin, 2000, 2003a, 2003b). These analyses suggest that gesture can compensate to some degree for verbal deficits (Fex & Månsson, 1998). However, the nature of this compensation varies markedly across aphasia types (Cicone, Wapner, Foldi, Zurif, & Gardner, 1979). Because AphasiaBank dialogues are collected in the same fashion across tasks we can make consistent assessments of the usage of gesture within and across these types.

The detailed analysis of gestural patterns can be very time consuming. Many analyses of gesture have focused on the nature of the synchrony between speech and gesture (Allen et al., 2007; McNeill, 1985). For analyses of this type, investigators often rely on linkage of speech to gesture through the Elan (http://www.lat-mpi.eu/tools/elan/) video annotator. The CLAN program called CHAT2ELAN converts AphasiaBank transcripts to Elan. Researchers can then analyse gesture–speech patterns inside Elan. Afterwards they can export the data back to CHAT, using the ELAN2CHAT program.

CLAN also provides its own methods for analysing gestures. These methods focus less on the synchrony between speech and gesture (although that can also be annotated) and more on the profiling of gestural sequences, as analysed in Kendon (1982). To briefly illustrate this approach, consider the sequence of gestures produced by participant adler11a. This 80-year-old male participant has severe Broca's aphasia (WAB AQ = 17) and is 12 years post-onset. Within the context of the AphasiaBank protocol this participant produced only the words *oh, no, well,* and *hello.* Yet, through his gestures, he was able to communicate about the following 19 events within the context of the retelling of the Cinderella story: shaking hands (indicating the start of the narrative), turning a page in the book (moving on to the next event), stepsisters playing (accompanied by singing to illustrate play), Cinderella sweeping (brushing on table), turns page, receiving invitation to ball (hand receives paper), Cinderella requesting to go (wanting expression and fingers indicating walking), stepmother refusing (head shake and word "no"), clothing selection (hands touch objects, followed by "well"), looking beautiful (smiles, looks up, and gasps at beauty), ripping of the dress (cross-body arm motions), throwing the dress away (tossing object across body and then forcefully to side), crying (head on arm, hand covers face, sobs), turns the page, being at the ball (dancing gestures with hands and body, sings tune from Disney movie), turns page, falling in love (gasps, hand to heart, head down, hugs), losing a shoe (object drops and hand reaches under table, gestures object slipping away), kissing goodbye, Prince knocks on door, waving hello, and kissing again. This entire sequence of 19 events was produced in a span of 49 seconds.

Figure 3 illustrates how these activities are coded in the CLAN transcript with a focus on the activities at line 721 describing the grabbing and ripping of Cinderella's dress. In the right hand side of this screenshot we see the basic CHAT transcript with codes like &=imit:ripping describing the ripping action (and sound effect) produced by the participant. In the bottom left we see the QuickTime video window, which can be controlled through links from the transcript or by the scroll buttons in that window. In the top left we see a text file called 5dress.cut, which analyses the sequence of gestures beginning at line 718. This breakout window focuses on the analysis of the eight segments of fifth gesture sequence, which are labelled as 5A-5B-5C-5D-5E-5F-5G-5H. Only the first two segments of the sequence are visible in the part of 5dress.cut shown here, but the others follow below those. Each gesture is then further analysed to indicate the dynamics of the action, the major body part involved, the classification of the gesture, and its functional meaning. The classification field uses keywords that can then be searched with FREQ.

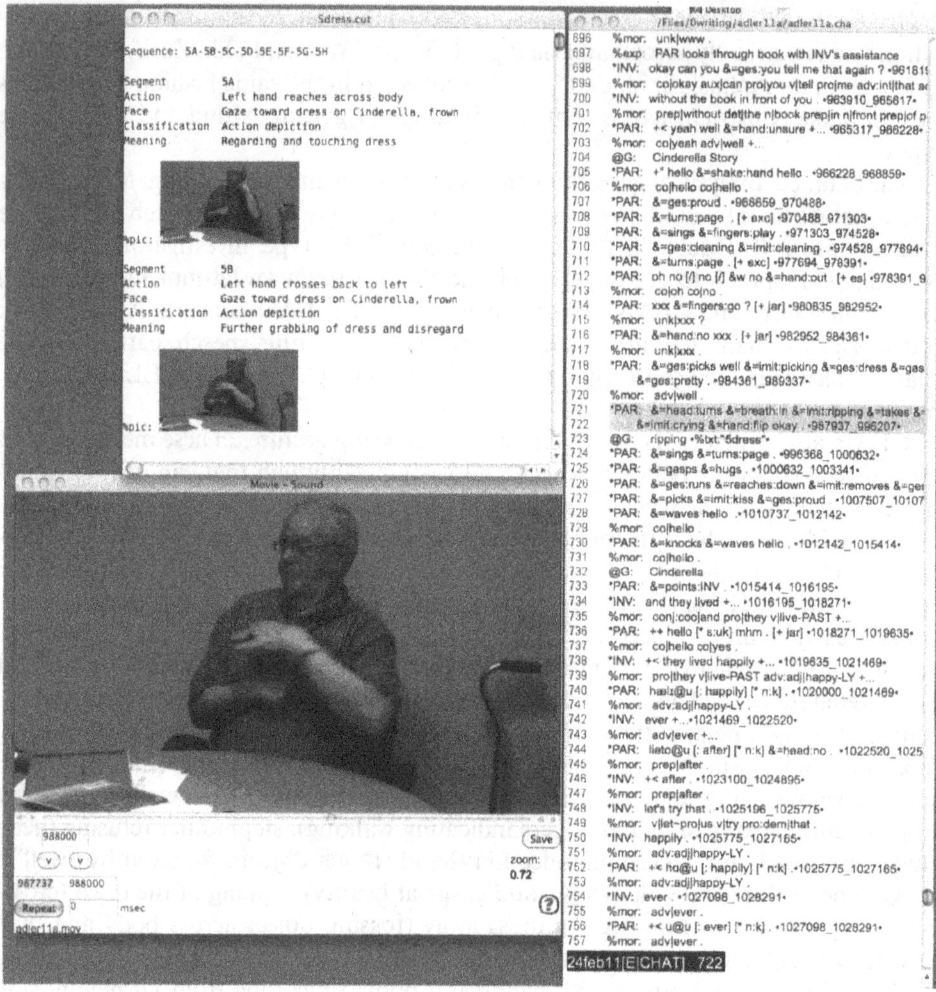

Figure 3. Transcript arrangement for gesture coding in CLAN.

Some of these gestures are produced as single gesture sequences with separate retraction and some are produced as parts of larger sequences. For each of these gesture sequences we then create a small separate small file link to the main transcript file. Here is an illustration of the breakout for the sequence in which the stepmother rips off and discards Cinderella's dress. The main transcript has this information:

*PAR: &=head:turns &=breath:in &=imit:ripping &=takes &=ges:away
&=imit:crying &=hand:flip okay.
@G: dress ripping sequence •%txt:"5dress"•

When the transcriber clicks on the bullet at the end of the @G line, a secondary file called 5dress.cut opens up. This file allows the transcriber to enter freeform coding of the gesture sequence. Here is a sample of the first few lines of this file:

@Media: adler11a, movie
Sequence: 5A-5B-5C-5D-5E-5F-5G-5H-5J-5K
Segment 5A

Action	Left hand reaches across body
Face	Gaze toward dress on Cinderella, frown
Classification	Action depiction
Meaning	Regarding and touching dress
%pic: •987737_988000•	
Segment	5B
Action	Left hand crosses back to left
Face	Gaze toward dress on Cinderella, frown
Classification	Action depiction
Meaning	Further grabbing of dress and disregard
%pic: •988000_988300•	

This file then continues with an analysis of the remaining eight segments of the dress-ripping sequence. When this file is opening up directly from the main file it displays the clips associated with the first frame of each segment given in the %pic lines. In general, this form of analysis allows us to understand the details of the ways in which this participant uses gesture to convey a rich understanding of the Cinderella story.

Phonological and temporal analyses

AphasiaBank data can be analysed for phonological and phonetic structures using the Phon program (http://childes.psy.cmu.edu/phon) that was developed to be compatible with CHAT and CLAN. Phon use IPA Unicode on the %pho line in CHAT files to encode the precise phonological form of utterances. Using this information it can also perform automatic syllabification and alignment with target phonological structures. The audio corresponding to individual utterances in CHAT can be sent to Praat (www.fon.hum.uva.nl/praat/) for further detailed phonetic analysis and the results can then be recaptured in Phon/CHAT files.

CLAN also provides the TIMEDUR program that can compute overall session length, the durations of individual utterances and the lengths of the pauses between utterances. Programs such as DIST, COOCCUR, KEYMAP, and CHAINS can be used to analyse various aspects of sequences in discourse structure.

FUTURE DIRECTIONS AND CONCLUSION

The goal of this paper has been to illustrate the ways in which AphasiaBank data can be used to address substantive issues in the study of aphasia. We have shown how many indices and analyses that were previously computed by hand can now be computed automatically and accurately using the CLAN programs. Moreover, unlike previous work, the data, procedures, and results for these analyses are now being made fully public and can therefore be replicated and even challenged by anyone in the scientific community. The illustrative studies presented here constitute only a small sampling of the studies that can be conducted with these data. Additional ideas for future studies using the AphasiaBank database are continually being generated and posted at a link on the home page of the AphasiaBank website.

As AphasiaBank moves into the future it will need to confront several interesting challenges. As we move to collect data from a wider variety of languages we will need to translate and revise the protocol to match local cultural expectations, as well as patterns of bilingualism. We will need to develop specific methods for best assessing the language abilities of participants with global aphasia. We will need to implement data collection procedures that will maximise our ability to include naturalistic conversational data in settings such as meal preparation, event planning, game playing, and other casual interactions. We will also need to apply AphasiaBank methods to study the impact of therapy treatments. Finally, as we move forward with this expansion of the database and the scope of AphasiaBank we will want to build new programs and new methods of analysis. Fortunately we can address these future challenges with confidence, knowing that we have already constructed an important new tool for the study of aphasia.

REFERENCES

Allen, S., Özyürek, A., Kita, S., Brown, A., Furman, R., Ishizuka, T., et al. (2007). Language-specific and universal influences on children's syntactic packaging of Manner and Path: A comparison of English, Japanese, and Turkish. *Cognition, 102*, 16–48.

Berndt, R., Wayland, S., Rochon, E., Saffran, E., & Schwartz, M. (2000). *Quantitative production analysis: A training manual for the analysis of aphasic sentence production*. Hove, UK: Psychology Press.

Brink, T. L., Yesavage, J. A., Lum, O., Heersema, P., Adey, M. B., & Rose, T. L. (1982). Screening tests for geriatric depression. *Clinical Gerontologist, 1*, 37–44.

Cicone, M., Wapner, W., Foldi, N., Zurif, E., & Gardner, H. (1979). The relation between gesture and language in aphasic communication. *Brain and Language, 8*, 324–349.

Fergadiotis, G., & Wright, H. (2011). Lexical diversity for adults with and without aphasia across discourse elicitation tasks. *Aphasiology, 25*(11), 1414–1430.

Fergadiotis, G., Wright, H., & Capilouto, G. J. (2011). Productive vocabulary across discourse types. *Aphasiology, 25*(10), 1261–1278.

Fex, B., & Månsson, A.-C. (1998). The use of gestures as a compensatory strategy in adults with acquired aphasia compared to children with specific language impairment (SLI). *Journal of Neurolinguistics, 11*, 191–206.

Fletcher, P., & Garman, M. (1988). LARSPing by numbers. *British Journal of Disorders of Communication, 23*, 309–321.

Folstein, M., Folstein, S., & Fanjiang, G. (2002). *Mini-mental State Examination*. Lutz, FL: Psychological Assessment Resources, Inc.

Fromm, D., Holland, A., Armstrong, B. C., Forbes, M., MacWhinney, B., Risko, A., et al. (2011). "Better but no cigar": Persons with aphasia speak about their speech. *Aphasiology, 25*(11), 1431–1447.

Glosser, G., Wiener, M., & Kaplan, E. (1986). Communicative gestures in aphasia. *Brain and Language, 27*, 345–359.

Goodwin, C. (2000). Gesture, aphasia, and interaction. In D. McNeill (Ed.), *Language and gesture* (pp. 84–98). Cambridge, UK: Cambridge University Press.

Goodwin, C. (Ed.). (2003a). Conversational frameworks for the accomplishment of meaning in aphasia. In *Conversation and brain damage* (pp. 90–116). Oxford, UK: Oxford University Press.

Goodwin, C. (Ed.). (2003b). *Conversation and brain damage*. Oxford, UK: Oxford University Press.

Grimes, N. (2005). *Walt Disney's Cinderella*. New York: Random House.

Holmes, D. I., & Singh, S. (1996). A stylometric analysis of conversational speech of aphasic patients. *Literary and Linguistic Computing, 11*, 133–140.

Kaplan, E., Goodglass, H., & Weintraub, S. (2001). *Boston Naming Test. Second edition*. Austin, TX: Pro-Ed.

Kendon, A. (1982). The study of gesture: Some observations on its history. *Recherches Sémiotiques/Semiotic Inquiry, 2*(1), 45–62.

Kertész, A. (2007). *Western Aphasia Battery*. San Antonio, TX: PsychCorp.

Lee, L. (1966). Developmental sentence types: A method for comparing normal and deviant syntactic development. *Journal of Speech and Hearing Disorders, 31*, 331–330.

MacWhinney, B. (1978). The acquisition of morphophonology. *Monographs of the Society for Research in Child Development, 43*, Whole no. 1, 1–123.

MacWhinney, B. (2000). *The CHILDES Project: Tools for analysing talk* (3rd ed.). Mahwah, NJ: Lawrence Erlbaum Associates Inc.

MacWhinney, B., Fromm, D., Holland, A., Forbes, M., & Wright, H. (2010). Automated analysis of the Cinderella story. *Aphasiology, 24*, 856–868.

Malvern, D. D., Richards, B. J., Chipere, N., & Purán, P. (2004). *Lexical diversity and language development.* New York: Palgrave Macmillan.

McNeill, D. (1985). So you think gestures are nonverbal? *Psychological Review*, *92*, 350–371.

Nicholas, L., & Brookshire, R. (1993). A system for quantifying the informativeness and efficiency of the connected speech of adults with aphasia. *Journal of Speech and Hearing Research*, *36*, 338–350.

Parisse, C., & Le Normand, M. T. (2000). Automatic disambiguation of the morphosyntax in spoken language corpora. *Behavior Research Methods, Instruments, and Computers*, *32*, 468–481.

Pinker, S. (1979). Formal models of language learning. *Cognition*, *7*, 217–283.

Rochon, E., Saffran, E., Berndt, R., & Schwartz, M. (2000). Quantitative analysis of aphasic sentence production: Further development and new data. *Brain and Language*, *72*, 193–218.

Sagae, K., Davis, E., Lavie, A., MacWhinney, B., & Wintner, S. (2010). Morphosyntactic annotation of CHILDES transcripts. *Journal of Child Language*, *37*, 705–729.

Sagae, K., Lavie, A., & MacWhinney, B. (2005). Automatic measurement of syntactic development in child language. *Proceedings of the 43rd Meeting of the Association for Computational Linguistics* (pp. 197–204). Ann Arbor, MI: ACL.

Scarborough, H. S. (1990). Index of productive syntax. *Applied Psycholinguistics*, *11*, 1–22.

Thompson, C. K. (2011). *Northwestern assessment of verbs and sentences – revised*. Manuscript in preparation. Evanston, IL: Northwestern University Press.

Wright, H., & Capilouto, G. J. (2009). Manipulating task instructions to change narrative discourse performance. *Aphasiology*, *23*, 1295–1308.

Wright, H. H., Silverman, S. W., & Newhoff, M. (2003). Measures of lexical diversity in aphasia. *Aphasiology*, *17*, 443–452.

APHASIOLOGY, 2011, 25 (11), 1308–1326

Discourse treatment for word retrieval impairment in aphasia: The story so far

Mary Boyle

Department of Communication Sciences & Disorders, Montclair State University, Bloomfield, NJ, USA

Background: Impairment-focused aphasia treatment has an ultimate goal of improving language production in connected speech and communication in daily life. Although impairment-based treatment has typically been carried out in words or sentences, investigations have begun to explore the efficacy of treatment during discourse production. Focusing treatment on an impaired linguistic process during discourse production is a complex and challenging endeavour.
Aims: This paper aims to review investigations of discourse treatment for word retrieval impairment in aphasia in order to identify and discuss variables that emerge as being important considerations in clinical practice and continued research.
Main Contribution: Seven investigations that applied treatments during structured discourse production to improve word retrieval in participants with aphasia were reviewed. Treatment methods used in the investigations included phonologic and orthographic cues, semantic feature analysis, contingency-based cueing hierarchies, and repeated conversational engagement. The discourse contexts used for treatment were structured conversations or structured narrative discourse. All investigations reported positive outcomes for improved word retrieval abilities. Although treated vocabulary items did not improve in all cases, improvements in general processes of word retrieval were reported. Focusing treatment on the linguistic process of word retrieval resulted in changes to discourse macrostructure, at least in terms of the informativeness of the discourse. When attitudes and perceptions of the participants with aphasia or of naïve judges were assessed, the outcomes were generally favourable. One investigation provided evidence that treatment in structured discourse was related to improved word retrieval in real-life conversations.
Conclusions: There are several promising discourse treatment approaches for word retrieval impairments in aphasia. Systematic analysis of changes in the macrolinguistic processes of discourse, in real-life conversations, and in the attitudes and perceptions of participants with aphasia and others in future discourse treatment studies would enhance our insights about their efficacy.

Keywords: Aphasia; Aphasia treatment; Discourse treatment; Word retrieval impairment.

There has been a great deal of activity in the past two decades in developing treatments at the discourse level for people with aphasia. These investigations reflect a variety of orientations to aphasia treatment. A review of the literature reveals two

Address correspondence to: Mary Boyle, PhD, CCC-SLP, BC-ANCDS, Department of Communication Sciences & Disorders, Montclair State University, 1515 Broad Street, Bloomfield, NJ 07003, USA. E-mail: boylem@mail.montclair.edu

http://dx.doi.org/10.1080/02687038.2011.596185

broad areas of concentration: treatments that focus on naturally occurring (real-life) conversations and those that focus on improving linguistic performance by treating within a structured discourse context. The treatments focused on real-life conversations are typically described as social approaches or as consequence-based treatments because they attempt to address the consequences of aphasia in an individual's life (Holland, 2008; Simmons-Mackie, Elman, Holland, & Damico, 2007; Thompson, & Worrall, 2008). Such treatments attempt to provide people with aphasia with communicative experiences that resemble natural communication in everyday social life in order to enhance communicative confidence (Simmons-Mackie et al., 2007).

The social approach to aphasia treatment is usually contrasted with impairment-based treatments, which focus on direct treatment of the language impairment (Thompson, & Worrall, 2008). Investigations of impairment-based treatments typically focus treatment and outcome measures at the word or sentence level, although recently many studies have assessed whether these treatments of more basic linguistic units result in changed discourse production (Boyle, 2004a; Boyle & Coelho, 1995; Cameron, Wambaugh, Wright, & Nessler, 2006; Coelho, McHugh, & Boyle, 2000; Edmonds, Nadeau, & Kiran, 2008; Faroqi-Shah & Virion, 2009; Rider, Wright, Marshall, & Page, 2008; Schwartz, Saffran, Fink, Myers, & Martin, 1994). In part because the changes in discourse have been inconsistent, investigators have developed treatments that require people with aphasia to work on specific linguistic skills (e.g., word retrieval or syntactic formulation) while they are producing discourses. The aim of these discourse treatments is to improve linguistic skills in communicative activities that are similar to, but more structured than, those used in everyday communication (Simmons-Mackie et al., 2007) in hopes of effecting change at a level that is likely to have a consequence in the person's everyday life.

Focusing treatment on a specific language process during discourse production is a complex and challenging endeavour. In addition to considering how to improve the targeted language process, investigators must consider the kind of discourse to use as a context for treating the language process, how to elicit a robust number of exemplars of the target process in the discourses, and how to measure the outcome of treatment. The aim of this paper is to explore some of these challenges and to review how they have been approached in investigations of discourse treatment for word retrieval impairment. The review is limited to data-based papers in English and to investigations that are focused on treatment that occurs at least in part during discourse production, with discourse-level outcomes reported. The review is also restricted to aphasia that is caused by stroke or traumatic brain injury; treatments for progressive aphasia are not included.

IMPAIRMENT-BASED DISCOURSE TREATMENT

Microlinguistic and macrolinguistic discourse impairments in aphasia

The microlinguistic structure of discourse (e.g., lexical and grammatical forms) is generally described as being more impaired by aphasia than its macrolinguistic structure (the conceptual, narrative, and pragmatic organisation of discourse) (Bloom, 1994; Davis, 2007; Glosser, 1993). Disruptions of the microlinguistic structure that have been reported to occur in the discourse of people with aphasia include lexical errors, syntactic errors, and reduced syntactic complexity (Glosser, 1993; Rochon, Saffran, Berndt, & Schwartz, 2000; Saffran, Berndt, & Schwartz, 1989).

Despite the fact that people with aphasia "can tell a good story" (Davis, 2007, p. 138), there is some evidence that the macrolinguistic structure of their discourse is affected by their microlinguistic impairments. The literature indicates that, compared to neurologically intact adults, people with aphasia omitted essential propositions, produced fewer propositions, and repeated propositions in discourses (Christiansen, 1995; Nicholas & Brookshire, 1995). Christiansen (1995) attempted to relate these macrolinguistic difficulties to the microlinguistic impairments. For example, she proposed that participants with anomic aphasia omitted entire propositions because of their word retrieval problems, and that this resulted in incomplete narratives. She suggested that participants with conduction aphasia produced multiple repetitions of entire propositions in their attempts to self-correct their paraphasic or paragrammatic errors. Other investigators have reported that people with aphasia produced incomplete cohesive ties and a limited range of connective forms compared to neurologically intact adults (see Bloom, 1994, for a review). Bloom suggested that these aphasic impairments contributed to the production of vague and ambiguous discourses. Impairment-based discourse treatment focuses on improving the microlinguistic impairments in order to improve the macrolinguistic processes underlying discourse construction and thus enhance communicative effectiveness.

Structured discourse versus real-life discourse

Adults typically use conversational discourse to communicate in their everyday lives, but the complexity of such real-life discourse can be a difficult context for impairment-based treatment. Within the conversational exchange of questions and comments, participants may tell their partners about events (narrative discourse), provide directions or instructions (procedural discourse), describe something in detail (descriptive discourse), or explain something in depth (expository discourse). In everyday conversations participants interrupt and overlap each other (i.e., there are no rigid turns) and they share control of topics (Simmons-Mackie et al., 2007). In real-life discourse speakers are free to switch between discourse types and to vary the specific words and syntactic structures that they use. This freedom poses a challenge when treatment is focused on specific linguistic impairments in discourse, because unless some structure is imposed on the discourse, the person with aphasia may not have many (or any) opportunities to produce the process that is targeted for improvement. For example, a real-life discourse might not contain any examples of a specific syntactic structure. Likewise, depending on the topic, the variety of nouns and verbs that are produced may be very limited, reducing the number of different words that need to be retrieved. In such cases the person with aphasia would not have many opportunities to practise the targeted language process. With little opportunity to practise, the likelihood that the process will improve is limited.

In order to evoke targeted processes frequently during treatment sessions, investigators employ structured discourse instead of real-life discourse. The "structure" of structured discourse typically includes limiting the discourse to one type, controlling the topic(s), allocating turns, and eliciting responses. In this way structured discourse is more similar to traditional impairment-based aphasia therapy than it is to real-life discourse. Another difference between structured discourse and real-life discourse is in the provision of feedback, correction, and evaluation by the clinician. This contrasts with real-life discourse, in which participants add comments or seek new information from partners rather than evaluating and correcting a partner's comment or response (Simmons-Mackie et al., 2007).

Evaluating outcomes of impairment-based discourse treatments

In order to assess the effects of impairment-based discourse treatment, the clinician must decide whether to evaluate changes at the microlinguistic level, the macrolinguistic level, or both. Microlinguistic analysis methods aim to measure change of the targeted linguistic process in discourse. Macrolinguistic measures are used to examine whether the organisation, structure, or pattern of discourse changes. Aside from speculations like those of Christiansen (1995) and Bloom (1994) cited earlier, there are few data available to assist clinicians and researchers in determining how specific changes at the microlinguistic level of discourse might affect its macrolinguistic structure. Therefore it is difficult to make an informed choice about which macrolinguistic measure might best capture a specific microlinguistic change.

The choice of microlinguistic analysis methods depends on the linguistic impairment that is the target of treatment. These methods might focus on lexical diversity (Rider et al., 2008), production of specific word types like nouns and verbs (Mayer & Murray, 2003), instances of word-finding difficulties (Boyle, 2004a; German, 1991), or analysis of morphological and syntactic production (Rochon et al., 2000; Saffran et al., 1989). The choice of macrolinguistic analysis methods is influenced by the type of discourse elicited. For narrative discourses, these methods might include assessing cohesion and coherence (Bloom, 1994; Glosser, 1993), quantifying the amount of information and the efficiency with which it is produced (Nicholas & Brookshire, 1993), assessing whether main concepts or essential propositions are conveyed (Christiansen, 1995; Joanette & Goulet, 1990; Nicholas & Brookshire, 1995), or analysing the global structure or story grammar (Ulatowska, Freedman-Stern, Doyel, Macaluso-Haynes, & North, 1983). For conversational discourse, macrolinguistic methods might include elements of conversation analysis (Oelschlager & Damico, 1998) or ethnographic methodology (Albright & Purves, 2008).

Because impairment-based discourse treatment studies apply treatment within the context of structured discourse production, it is not surprising that outcomes are also assessed in structured discourse. However, improvement in structured discourse may not necessarily result in changes in real-life discourse given the differences between these two communication activities. Investigations vary in terms of what outcomes are assessed and in terms of the methods chosen to assess them. This variability across investigations is probably related, at least in part, to the exploratory nature of impairment-based discourse treatment studies. These treatments are still in the discovery stage of clinical outcome research; that is, the treatment approaches are being developed, refined, and assessed to determine whether they show promise of being efficacious (Cherney, Patterson, Raymer, Frymark, & Schooling, 2008; Robey, 2004). During this period of exploration, some investigators have concentrated solely on assessing whether the targeted linguistic process improves without assessing any other outcomes. Other investigators have also assessed whether there are changes beyond the linguistic process; for example, they tried to determine whether there were associated changes at the macrolinguistic level, in real-life discourse, in other aspects of life participation, or in the attitudes of the participants toward their communicative abilities. This variation is understandable at this early stage of research. It does, however, make it difficult to predict whether a particular treatment approach is likely to have consequences beyond the discourse task used in the treatment study.

Discourse treatments for word retrieval

Table 1 lists studies that have targeted word retrieval in discourse treatment. Seven investigations, all single-participant designs or case reports, involved 16 participants with a variety of aphasia types. The most commonly used discourse contexts for treatment were structured conversation and narrative discourse. All investigations assessed outcomes in structured discourse. Other outcome measures varied across the investigations.

Phonologic and orthographic cueing. Two investigations used phonologic and orthographic cues in treatment (Greenwood, Grassly, Hickin, & Best, 2010; Herbert, Best, Hickin, Howard, & Osborne, 2003). In both instances the investigators added structured conversational tasks to the study design after discovering that word retrieval improvements made in single-word confrontation naming tasks did not generalise to word retrieval in structured discourse. During the discourse phase of treatment in these studies, phonologic and orthographic cues were provided to assist in word retrieval as necessary while the participants engaged in two structured conversational tasks. The first was a barrier task, which is essentially a structured conversational exchange that constrains the topics and the forms of the interchanges (i.e., the participant attempts to communicate the name of a hidden stimulus to the investigator). The second task was a structured conversational exchange about a topic related to the vocabulary items that were targeted in treatment.

Although the two investigations used similar treatment strategies, the microlinguistic outcomes that they assessed were different. Herbert and colleagues (2003) assessed microlinguistic changes in structured conversation and reported that none of the six participants improved their production of treated nouns. The investigators noted that although production of the treated nouns did not improve, the participants' responses in structured conversation were more communicatively appropriate after treatment because they were "able to access vocabulary that explained their needs or thoughts more effectively" (pp. 1176–1177). It appears, then, that even though the target vocabulary items did not improve, some general process of word retrieval ability did improve.

Greenwood and colleagues (2010) assessed microlinguistic changes in a structured narrative discourse (the Cinderella story) rather than in a structured conversational task similar to the one used in treatment. They reported that the participant did not significantly improve on a measure of word retrieval in structured narrative discourse. These investigators also assessed whether the participant's word retrieval changed during real-life conversations with his usual conversational partner. To do this they asked the participant and his partner to record 10 minutes of natural conversation (without topic restrictions) in their home. They analysed the middle 5 minutes of the sample using procedures reported in Herbert, Hickin, Howard, Osborne, and Best (2008), which assess content word production and content word errors. The participant's production of content words in the real-life conversations improved after treatment and this improvement was maintained after treatment was withdrawn. The occurrence of content word errors in the real-life conversations decreased after treatment, but returned to pre-discourse-treatment levels at follow-up.[1]

[1] Herbert and colleagues (2003) reported that they also assessed microlinguistic changes in the Cinderella narrative and in real-life conversations, but they did not report the results in their paper.

TABLE 1
Summary of investigations targeting spoken word retrieval with discourse treatment

Investigation	*Number of participants*	*Aphasia type*	*Treatment*	*Outcomes: Word/sentence level*	*Outcomes: Structured discourse*	*Outcomes: Real-life discourse*	*Outcomes: Life participation, personal identity/attitude/feelings*
PHONOLOGIC/ORTHOGRAPHIC CUEING							
Herbert, Best, Hickin, Howard, & Osborne (2003)	6	3: Broca's 2: Anomic 1: Wernicke's	*Phase 1*: Noun picture naming, half of targets treated with phonologic cues and distractors and half with orthographic cues and distractors provided in a contingency-based hierarchy, beginning with minimal information and adding phonemes or letters until the item was named or the whole word had been presented for repetition; 50 items never treated *Phase 2*: Tasks designed to systematically move from picture naming toward conversational speech with same stimuli as Phase 1: naming to definition, PACE activity (*structured conversation*), producing spoken lists of treated items in goal-directed categories, using treated words in *structured conversation*	*Phase 1*: 1 participant improved naming of treated and untreated items, 4 improved naming of treated but not untreated items,1 did not improve *Phase 2*: 5 improved naming of treated but not untreated items, 1 did not improve *Maintenance*: All participants maintained improvement 8 weeks after treatment withdrawn	*Structured conversation*: *Phase 1:* Not assessed *Phase 2:* No improvement on target nouns, all participants improved communicative appropriateness of responses (change for 1 participant was statistically significant) *Maintenance:* Not reported *Narrative discourse*: Cinderella re-tell: Results not reported in paper	*Conversation with friend or relative*: Results not reported in paper	*Communication views questionnaire*: Authors questioned reliability of instrument; provided responses for only one participant

(*Continued*)

TABLE 1
(Continued)

Investigation	*Number of participants*	*Aphasia type*	*Treatment*	*Outcomes: Word/sentence level*	*Outcomes: Structured discourse*	*Outcomes: Real-life discourse*	*Outcomes: Life participation, personal identity/attitude/feelings*
Greenwood, Grassly, Hickin, & Best (2010)	1	Anomia	*Phase 1:* 60 nouns for picture naming using combined phonologic and orthographic cues with up to 3 distractors; 60 items using combined phonologic and orthographic cues without distractors; both conditions provided in a contingency-based hierarchy as above; 50 items presented every session for naming but no cueing; 50 items presented only in probe sessions *Phase 2:* Same as Phase 2 in Herbert et al. (2003) above, with an additional set of 75 multisyllabic nouns added to stimuli	*Phase 1*: Improved naming of treated and untreated items *Phase 2*: No additional improvement of any items from Phase 1, but multisyllabic words introduced in this phase improved *Maintenance:* Improvements maintained 8 weeks after treatment withdrawn	*Narrative discourse*: Cinderella re-tell: No change	*Conversation with usual conversational partner*: Increase in content words and decrease in content word errors *Maintenance*: Increase in content words maintained 8 weeks after treatment withdrawn	*Communication Disability Profile*[a]: Improved scores in activities, participation, and emotional consequences

SEMANTIC FEATURE ANALYSIS							
Boyle (2004)	3	Conduction Broca's Broca's	*C-SFA:* Naming of 10 pictured nouns while clinician systematically guided participants to produce semantic features associated with target, features written on chart as they were produced; 10 pictured nouns reserved for probes *D-SFA:* Participants produced *narrative discourses* about progressively longer picture sequences (26 wordless comic strips and 7 wordless picture books); same feature generation production and cueing as above, but only when participants could not produce a noun while telling the stories	All participants Improved naming of treated and untreated nouns *Maintenance*: Improvements maintained 1 month after treatment withdrawn	*Narrative discourse*: All participants increased the number of correct information units 2 participants increased the percentage of correct information units 1 participant reduced the percentage of nouns evidencing retrieval difficulty *Maintenance*: Improvements maintained 1 month after treatment withdrawn	Not assessed	Naïve raters considered one participant to demonstrate better word retrieval, convey more information, and communicate more efficiently after than before treatment

(*Continued*)

TABLE 1
(Continued)

Investigation	*Number of participants*	*Aphasia type*	*Treatment*	*Outcomes: Word/sentence level*	*Outcomes: Structured discourse*	*Outcomes: Real-life discourse*	*Outcomes: Life participation, personal identity/attitude/feelings*
Antonucci (2009)	2	Conduction Anomic	*Group treatment.* 2 sessions: C-SFA treatment as outlined above in Boyle (2004) *Structured conversation:* 12 sessions: modified PACE procedure – participants took turns describing increasingly complex picture stimuli that other could not see, using SFA cueing when participants could not produce a word	No improvement in confrontation noun naming	*Narrative discourse:* Both participants increased the percentage of nouns retrieved Both participants increased the number of correct information units in discourse 1 participant increased correct information units produced per minute *Maintenance*: Both participants maintained improvements 6 weeks after treatment withdrawn	Not assessed	Unsolicited anecdotal self-reports of improved word retrieval in daily communication

Peach & Reuter (2010)	2	Anomic	Participants described pictured scenes depicting two or more events *(narrative discourse)* and answered procedural questions *(procedural discourse)*. Following discourse production, clinician selected failed lexical items from discourses and used C-SFA treatment as outlined above in Boyle (2004), but targeting both nouns and verbs	Both participants improved confrontation naming of untreated nouns and verbs *Maintenance:* Improvements maintained 4.5 months after treatment withdrawn	*Narrative discourse:* Both participants improved verbal productivity (number of words per T-unit) and informativeness (percentage of correct information units) Neither participant reduced word-finding behaviors *Maintenance:* Participant 1 maintained improved productivity 4.5 months after treatment withdrawn; Participant 2 not available for follow-up	Not assessed	Not assessed

(*Continued*)

TABLE 1
(Continued)

Investigation	*Number of participants*	*Aphasia type*	*Treatment*	*Outcomes: Word/sentence level*	*Outcomes: Structured discourse*	*Outcomes: Real-life discourse*	*Outcomes: Life participation, personal identity/attitude/feelings*
OTHER BARRIER TASK TREATMENT PARADIGMS							
Goral & Kempler (2009)	1	Nonfluent aphasia	Sentence repetition Sentence reading *Structured conversation*: Modified constraint-induced aphasia treatment: participant constrained to use verbal communication containing a verb during informative verbal exchanges: card games, script generation, picture description, story co-construction, video recounts); requirements for participant's responses progressed from words/phrases to sentences to narratives; clinician used contingency-based cueing hierarchy if no verb was produced	Not assessed	*Narrative discourse:* Increased number of words produced per narrative, percentage of verbs produced per narrative, and verb-noun ratio, but not percentage of nouns produced *Maintenance*: Improvements maintained 10 weeks after treatment withdrawn	Not assessed	Naïve raters judged post-treatment narratives more favourably

Hengst, Duff, & Prior (2008); Hengst, Duff, & Dettmar (2010)	1	Anomic with severe memory impairment	*Semi-structured conversation*: Barrier task protocol: Clinician and participant worked together to place twelve target cards in identical arrangements on their playing boards through collaborative verbal referencing, which involves conversational repetition of card labels within and across sessions, while unable to view each other's boards. Focus was on repeated engagement rather than repeated behaviour	Not assessed	*Semi-structured conversation:* Improved labelling of all treated items	Not assessed	Not assessed

[a]Swinburn and Byng (2006).

The microlinguistic outcomes reported by these two investigations suggest that improvements made in one kind of discourse task (e.g., structured conversation), won't necessarily result in improvements in a different kind of discourse task (e.g., structured narrative discourse). They also suggest that production of specific vocabulary items targeted in treatment may not improve in probe tasks. However, there may be a general improvement in the word retrieval process of participants in discourse tasks that are similar to those used in treatment.

Neither Herbert et al. (2003) nor Greenwood et al. (2010) assessed macrolinguistic discourse changes, but both assessed changes in the participants' views about their ability to communicate. Herbert and colleagues expressed dissatisfaction with the reliability of the attitude questionnaire that they used and, although they reported results for one of the participants, the investigators stated that they did not feel that it was a useful outcome measure. Greenwood and colleagues used a published measure of activities, participation, and attitude (Swinburn & Byng, 2006) and reported that the participant's ratings of his activity, participation, and emotions improved after treatment.

Semantic feature analysis. Three investigations (Antonucci, 2009; Boyle, 2004b; Peach & Reuter, 2010) employed variations of semantic feature analysis (SFA) (Boyle, 2010) as a treatment in discourse. The investigations by Boyle (2004b) and by Peach and Reuter used sequential and complex pictures, respectively, to elicit structured narrative discourses. Whereas Boyle applied SFA immediately during the narrative production when a participant failed to retrieve a noun, Peach and Reuter applied SFA to problematic nouns after the participants finished producing the discourse. Antonucci used SFA procedures in group rather than in individual treatment. During the group sessions, participants performed PACE barrier-task activities using increasingly complex picture stimuli and narrative retells of fairytales and movie plots. Thus, the participants produced structured narrative discourses within the structured conversational discourse of the barrier task.

All three of these investigations assessed microlinguistic- and macrolinguistic-level outcomes using the stimuli developed by Nicholas and Brookshire (2003) to elicit structured narrative and procedural discourses. At the microlinguistic level, the investigators assessed changes in word retrieval in different ways. Antonucci (2009) examined the percentage of nouns produced, which increased for both participants after treatment. Neither of the other two investigations assessed this variable. Peach and Reuter (2010) assessed verbal productivity in terms of the number of words produced per T-unit. They reported that both participants improved on this measure after treatment. Neither of the other two investigations assessed this variable. Both Boyle (2004b) and Peach and Reuter (2010) assessed whether behaviours associated with word-finding trouble decreased. There was a positive outcome for only one of five participants (Boyle, 2004b). Although the microlinguistic measures varied across the investigations, it is worth noting that all of them employed general measures of word retrieval rather than examining for improvement of the specific vocabulary items that were targeted in treatment. As was the case with the phonologic and orthographic cueing studies of discourse treatment, the outcomes for these general measures of word retrieval were positive.

To assess change at the macrolinguistic level, all three investigations (Antonucci, 2008; Boyle, 2004b; Peach & Reuter, 2010) used measures of information content developed by Nicholas and Brookshire (2003). All participants in all of the studies increased production of informational content in some way, although the exact measures that improved varied among participants. Two of three participants in Boyle's study, one of two participants in Antonucci's study, and both participants in Peach and Reuter's study increased the percentage of correct information units (CIUs) in their discourses. Antonucci and Boyle reported that all participants increased the number of correct information units produced during discourse; Peach and Reuter did not assess this measure. One of two participants in Antonucci's study produced more CIUs per minute after treatment; neither of the other investigations assessed this variable. In summary, at the macrolinguistic level, all of the investigations reported improvements in informativeness of structured narrative discourses following treatment. The fact that not all participants demonstrated changes on the same informativeness measures may be related to participant factors such as type and severity of aphasia or pattern of word retrieval breakdown, or it may be related to the fact that not all of the investigations reported all of the informativeness measures.

None of the investigations assessed changes in real-life discourse, although Antonucci (2010) reported unsolicited anecdotes indicating that one participant improved word retrieval in daily communication. Boyle reported that naïve judges rated one of three participants as more successful in finding and saying the correct words after treatment. This was the same participant whose word-finding behaviours decreased after treatment, a fact that will be discussed in more detail later.

Thus it appears that SFA narrative discourse treatment for word retrieval impairment was associated with improvements in informativeness of the discourses at the macrostructural level. The exact components of informational content that improved varied among the participants. This highlights the importance of systematically examining this relationship in future investigations so that we can better understand how the nature and/or severity of the microlinguistic impairments influence the macrostructure of the discourses that are produced.

Other barrier task treatment paradigms. Two investigations employed the structured conversational exchanges of barrier tasks to treat word retrieval, but they used markedly different treatment approaches within these tasks. Goral and Kempler (2009) modified constraint-induced aphasia treatment procedures to target verb retrieval. Their treatment tasks progressed from the typical request–response card games of the constraint-induced treatment protocol to narrative discourse tasks like story co-construction. When the participant had difficulty producing a verb, the researcher provided a contingency-based cueing hierarchy. After treatment, the participant improved on microlinguistic measures (total number of words, percentage of verbs, and verb–noun ratios) in structured narratives. This provides another instance, like those reported in the phonologic-orthographic cueing studies and in the SFA studies, in which measures of general word retrieval ability showed positive changes after discourse treatment. Macrolinguistic discourse outcomes were not assessed. Naïve judges rated post-treatment narratives more favourably than pre-treatment narratives on a social-communicative effectiveness questionnaire, suggesting that the discourse-level verb treatment was associated with language changes that positively affected the perception of the participant's communication.

In another barrier-task discourse treatment for word retrieval, Hengst and colleagues (Hengst, Duff, & Dettmar, 2010; Hengst, Duff, & Prior, 2008) required the participant and the clinician to collaborate in constructing verbal labels for people and places in a semi-structured conversation task that focused on repeated engagement.

In this paradigm, although the topic of conversation was constrained, production of the labels was permitted to vary freely as it does in real-life conversational repetition, thus allowing natural convergence to agreed-upon labels across the treatment sessions rather than requiring repetition of the same label in each session. The participant, who had a severe memory impairment in addition to anomic aphasia, improved his ability to use the co-constructed labels for all treated items at the end of treatment. The investigators did not assess macrolinguistic discourse changes or report effects of improved labelling in the participant's everyday life. This was an exploratory study designed to assess whether this non-traditional approach to treating word retrieval impairment was a viable option. The positive outcome suggests that it is. However, its potential efficacy as a treatment method would be even more evident if information about outcomes in discourse situations other than the treatment task had been reported. This kind of information might attract clinicians and other investigators to explore the repeated engagement approach in their own work.

DISCUSSION AND CONCLUSIONS

Seven investigations applied treatments during structured discourse production to improve word retrieval in participants with aphasia. Treatment methods included phonologic and orthographic cues, semantic feature analysis, contingency-based cueing hierarchies, and repeated conversational engagement. Although conclusions about treatment efficacy are premature at this point in the research process, some preliminary observations might be useful for clinicians and researchers to consider as treatment research in this area moves forward.

Discourse treatment for word retrieval impairment can improve word retrieval in discourse

All investigations that assessed microlinguistic changes relating to improved word retrieval abilities reported positive outcomes (Antonucci, 2009; Goral & Kempler, 2009; Greenwood et al., 2010; Hengst et al., 2008, 2010; Herbert et al., 2003; Peach & Reuter, 2010). Interestingly, the vocabulary items targeted in treatment were not necessarily the items that improved on these outcome measures. Hengst and colleagues reported that the participant in their investigation improved his ability to produce the labels that were the focus of treatment, but they only assessed this outcome in the treatment task, not in other discourse situations. Herbert and colleagues, in contrast, reported that participants' ability to produce the treated nouns did not improve in other structured conversational discourse tasks after treatment. These investigators noted, however, that participants' responses were more communicatively appropriate after treatment, and they attributed this to improved ability to access other vocabulary items. The remaining investigators who assessed microlinguistic outcomes used measures that were reflective of a generalised improvement in word retrieval abilities rather than improved retrieval of specific vocabulary items. These measures included the total number of words, the number of content words, the percentage of nouns or verbs, the number of words per T-unit, and the verb-to-noun ratio. The outcomes reported by these investigators suggest that the discourse treatments were improving the *process* of word retrieval rather than improving the ability to name specific items. Certainly this is a desired outcome for the participants with aphasia, since improvement of the process rather than of specific vocabulary items should be the primary goal of treatment to improve word retrieval. For clinicians and researchers, these results suggest that stimuli to assess outcomes need not be constrained to include treated vocabulary items as long as measures that capture changes in the general process of word retrieval are used.

Discourse treatment for word retrieval impairment does not necessarily result in long-lasting reduction in overt manifestations of word retrieval difficulty

Although one might suppose that overt evidence of word retrieval difficulties would decrease as word retrieval abilities improved, this was not always the case. Three investigations assessed behaviours that signalled word retrieval difficulties such as paraphasias, delays, and empty words. Greenwood and colleagues (2010) reported that the proportion of content words signalling word retrieval difficulty decreased following discourse treatment but returned to pre-discourse-treatment levels at the follow-up probe. Boyle (2004b) assessed the percentage of T-units that contained evidence of word retrieval difficulty and reported that they decreased for one of three participants after discourse treatment. Peach and Reuter (2010) assessed the number of word-finding behaviours per T-unit and reported that they did not decrease for either participant as a result of treatment. In fact, Peach and Reuter reported that for one participant, as more words were retrieved throughout the treatment period, more behaviours that signalled word-finding trouble were produced as well. Because two of the investigations achieved limited success in reducing overt manifestations of lexical retrieval difficulties, it appears that these behaviours are amenable to change. There is some evidence that reduction of these behaviours might influence the perception of word retrieval ability, at least in naïve judges: the only participant in Boyle's investigation rated as better at finding and saying the right words after treatment was the sole participant whose overt manifestations of word retrieval difficulty decreased. Thus it might be useful to target the reduction of behaviours that signal word retrieval problems if these contribute to negative perceptions about a speaker's abilities. Assessment of this outcome in future investigations could provide valuable information and insights in this regard.

Focusing discourse treatment on microlinguistic impairments can change the macrolinguistic processes of discourse

Three investigations (Antonucci, 2009; Boyle, 2004b; Peach & Reuter, 2010) reported that aspects of informativeness improved as a result of discourse treatment for word retrieval impairment. Five of seven participants in the semantic feature analysis treatment studies increased the percentage of correct, informative words in their discourses. None of the seven investigations reviewed in this paper, however, assessed other macrolinguistic discourse changes. Apart from speculation by a few investigators (Bloom, 1994; Christiansen, 1995), there are few data to help us understand whether or how reducing the severity of a specific linguistic impairment like word retrieval impairment will improve the conceptual, narrative, or pragmatic organisation of discourse. Systematic collection and analysis of such data would provide valuable information about whether impairment-based treatment affects more global aspects of communicative effectiveness.

Discourse treatment for word retrieval impairments can change the attitudes and perceptions of the participants with aphasia and of others

One investigation used a published tool to solicit the participant's views about how the treatment had affected his life and attitude (Greenwood et al., 2010), two obtained social-validation ratings from naïve judges (Boyle, 2004b; Goral & Kempler, 2009), and one reported unsolicited anecdotal observations from the participants (Antonucci, 2009). Most of these outcomes reported positive changes in attitudes and perceptions, the exception being the lack of perceived change in word-finding behaviours for two of the three participants in Boyle's investigation. Kagan and colleagues (2008) reported that policy makers and funding sources recommend the use of patient-reported outcomes when assessing the effects of treatment. Cupit, Rochon, Leonard, and Laird (2010) suggest that social validation measures may serve as proxy measurements for participants' success in interacting with community members. Both forms of outcome measures have the potential to provide information about the impact of treatment on the everyday life of participants with aphasia. Positive results on such measures reinforce the value of a treatment. Negative results on such measure may indicate ways in which the treatment can be modified to improve its effect on everyday functioning.

There is some evidence that discourse treatment for word retrieval impairment can improve word retrieval in real-life conversations

Only one of seven investigations formally assessed change in real-life conversations (Greenwood et al., 2010). One other investigation (Antonucci, 2009) reported unsolicited anecdotes from participants or family members that the improvements seen in treatment were affecting the participants' everyday communication. If real-life change is our ultimate treatment goal we must become more diligent about assessing it systematically. It is understandable that few investigators are able to spend time observing participants in their daily lives. However, there are other means of accomplishing this kind of assessment, as demonstrated by Greenwood and colleagues (2010). They asked the participant to record conversations with a regular communication partner in his home. This method was not without its pitfalls: the investigators reported that they had to exclude one of the real-life conversations from analysis because when they listened to it they discovered that it was actually more of a monologue than a conversation. Nevertheless, they succeeded in gathering enough real-life conversations to demonstrate a positive change in them. Routinely adding such a procedure to discourse treatment investigations and clinical practice might be an efficient way to extend outcome assessments to participants' daily lives. This would add significantly to our knowledge about the actual life consequences of our treatments. In whatever way it is accomplished, functional performance in actual life situations needs to be assessed in order to understand whether and how our treatments are actually affecting the daily lives of our clients and research participants. This would be the strongest possible evidence that treatment makes a difference.

REFERENCES

Albright, E., & Purves, B. (2008). Exploring SentenceShaper™: Treatment and augmentative possibilities. *Aphasiology, 22*, 741–752.

Antonucci, S. M. (2009). Use of semantic feature analysis in group aphasia treatment. *Aphasiology, 23*, 854–866.

Bloom, R. L. (1994). Hemispheric responsibility and discourse production: Contrasting patients with unilateral left and right hemisphere damage. In R. L. Bloom, L. K. Obler, S. DeSanti, & J. S. Ehrlich (Eds.), *Discourse analysis and applications: Studies in adults clinical populations* (pp. 81–94). Hillside, NJ: Lawrence Erlbaum Associates.

Boyle, M. (2004a). Semantic feature analysis treatment for anomia in two fluent aphasia syndromes. *American Journal of Speech-Language Pathology, 13*, 236–249.

Boyle, M. (2004b). *Discourse treatment for word retrieval impairment in chronic aphasia*. Paper presented at the 34th Clinical Aphasiology Conference, Park City, UT, May.

Boyle, M. (2010). Semantic feature analysis treatment for aphasic word retrieval impairments: What's in a name? *Topics in Stroke Rehabilitation, 17*, 411–422.

Boyle, M., & Coelho, C. A. (1995). Application of semantic feature analysis as a treatment for aphasic dysnomia. *American Journal of Speech-Language Pathology, 4*, 94–98.

Cameron, R. M., Wambaugh, J. L., Wright, S. M., & Nessler, C. L. (2006). Effects of a combined semantic/phonologic cueing treatment on word retrieval in discourse. *Aphasiology, 20*, 269–285.

Cherney, L. R., Patterson, J. P., Raymer, A., Frymark, T., & Schooling, T. (2008). Evidence-based systematic review: Effects of intensity of treatment and constraint-induced language therapy for individuals with stroke-induced aphasia. *Journal of Speech, Language, and Hearing Research, 5*, 1282–1299.

Christiansen, J. A. (1995). Coherence violations and propositional usage in the narratives of fluent aphasics. *Brain and Language, 51*, 291–317.

Coelho, C. A., McHugh, R. E., & Boyle, M. (2000). Semantic feature analysis as a treatment for aphasic dysnomia: A replication. *Aphasiology, 14*, 133–142.

Cupit, J., Rochon, E., Leonard, C., & Laird, L. (2010). Social validation as a measure of improvement after aphasia treatment: Its usefulness and influencing factors. *Aphasiology, 24*, 1486–1500.

Davis, G. A. (2007). *Aphasiology: Disorders and clinical practice* (2nd ed.). Boston, MA: Allyn & Bacon.

Edmonds, L. A., Nadeau, S. E., & Kiran, S. (2008). Effect of Verb Network Strengthening Treatment (VNeST) on lexical retrieval of content words in sentences in persons with aphasia. *Aphasiology, 23*, 402–424.

Faroqi-Shah, Y., & Virion, C. R. (2009). Constraint-induced language therapy for agrammatism: Role of grammaticality restraints. *Aphasiology, 23*, 977–988.

German, D. J. (1991). *Test of word finding in discourse (TWFD): Administration, scoring, interpretation, and technical manual*. Austin, TX: Pro-Ed.

Glosser, G. (1993). Discourse production patterns in neurologically impaired and aged populations. In H. H. Brownell & Y. Joanette (Eds.), *Narrative discourse in neurologically impaired and normal aging adults* (pp. 191–211). San Diego, CA: Singular.

Goral, M., & Kempler, D. (2009). Training verb production in communicative context: Evidence from a person with chronic non-fluent aphasia. *Aphasiology, 23*, 1383–1397.

Greenwood, A., Grassly, J., Hickin, J., & Best, W. (2010). Phonological and orthographic cueing therapy: A case of generalised improvement. *Aphasiology, 24*, 991–1016.

Hengst, J. A., Duff, M. C., & Dettmer, A. (2010). Rethinking repetition in therapy: Repeated engagement as the social ground of learning. *Aphasiology, 24*, 887–901.

Hengst, J. A., Duff, M. C., & Prior, P. A. (2008). Multiple voices in clinical discourse and as clinical intervention. *International Journal of Language & Communcation Disorders, 43*, 58–68.

Herbert, R., Best, W., Hickin, J., Howard, D., & Osborne, F. (2003). Combining lexical and interactional approaches to therapy for word finding deficits in aphasia. *Aphasiology, 17*, 1163–1186.

Herbert, R., Hickin, J., Howard, D., Osborne, F., & Best, W. (2008). Do picture-naming tests provide a valid assessment of lexical retrieval in conversation in aphasia? *Aphasiology, 22*, 184–203.

Holland, A. L. (2008). Recent advances and future directions in aphasia therapy. *Brain Impairment, 9*, 179–190.

Joanette, Y., & Goulet, P. (1990). Narrative discourse in right-brain-damaged right-handers. In Y. Joanette & H. H. Brownell (Eds.), *Discourse ability and brain damage: Theoretical and empirical perspectives* (pp. 131–153). New York: Springer-Verlag.

Kagan, A., Simmons-Mackie, N., Rowland, A., Huijbregts, M., Shumway, E., McEwen, S., et al. (2008). Counting what counts: A framework for capturing real-life outcomes of aphasia intervention. *Aphasiology, 22*, 258–280.

Mayer, J. F., & Murray, L. L. (2003). Functional measures of naming in aphasia: Word retrieval in confrontation naming versus connected speech. *Aphasiology, 17*, 481–497.

Nicholas, L. E., & Brookshire, R. H. (1993). A system for quantifying the informativeness and efficiency of the connected speech of adults with aphasia. *Journal of Speech and Hearing Research, 36*, 338–351.

Nicholas, L. E., & Brookshire, R. H. (1995). Presence, completeness, and accuracy of main concepts in the connected speech of non-brain-damaged adults and adults with aphasia. *Journal of Speech and Hearing Research, 38*, 145–156.

Oelschlager, M., & Damico, J.S. (1998). Joint productions as a conversational strategy in aphasia. *Clinical Linguistics and Phonetics, 12*, 459–480.

Peach, R. K., & Reuter, K. A. (2010). A discourse-based approach to semantic feature analysis for the treatment of aphasic word retrieval failures. *Aphasiology, 24*, 971–990.

Rider, J. D., Wright, H. H., Marshall, R. C., & Page, J. L. (2008). Using semantic feature analysis to improve contextual discourse in adults with aphasia. *American Journal of Speech-Language Pathology, 17*, 161–172.

Robey, R. R. (2004). A five-phase model for clinical-outcome research. *Journal of Communication Disorders, 37*, 401–411.

Rochon, E., Saffran, E. M., Berndt, R. S., & Schwartz, M. F. (2000). Quantitative analysis of aphasic sentence production: Further development and new data. *Brain and Language, 72*, 193–218.

Saffran, E. M., Berndt, R. S., & Schwartz, M. F. (1989). The quantitative analysis of agrammatic production: Procedure and data. *Brain and Language, 37*, 440–479.

Schwartz, M. F., Saffran, E. M., Fink, R. B., Myers, J. L., & Martin, N. (1994). Mapping therapy: A treatment programme for agrammatism. *Aphasiology, 8*, 19–54.

Simmons-Mackie, N., Elman, R. J., Holland, A. L., & Damico, J. S. (2007). Management of discourse in group therapy for aphasia. *Topics in Language Disorders, 27*, 5–23.

Swinburn, K., & Byng, S. (2006). *The Communication Disabilities Profile*. London: Connect.

Thompson, C. K., & Worrall, L. (2008). Approaches to aphasia treatment. In N. Martin, C. K. Thompson, & L. Worrall (Eds.), *Aphasia rehabilitation: The impairment and its consequences*. San Diego, CA: Plural Publishing.

Ulatowska, H. K., Freedman-Stern, R., Doyel, A. W., Macaluso-Haynes, S., & North, A. J. (1983). Production of narrative discourse in aphasia. *Brain and Language, 19*, 317–334.

APHASIOLOGY, 2011, 25 (11), 1327–1346

A comparison of drill- and communication-based treatment for aphasia

Daniel Kempler[1] and Mira Goral[2]

[1]Communication Sciences and Disorders, Emerson College, Boston, MA, USA
[2]Speech-Language-Hearing Sciences, Lehman College, The City University of New York, NY, USA

Background: Traditional aphasia therapy is based primarily on repetition and drill. Recent treatment studies have suggested that communication-based interactions may be at least as effective if not more so in achieving positive outcomes.
Aims: This study was undertaken to directly compare the outcomes of drill-based vs. communication-based interactions in modified Constraint-Induced Aphasia Therapy.
Methods & Procedures: Two women with chronic non-fluent aphasia participated sequentially in two distinct treatment protocols designed to improve verb production in sentences. Both treatment protocols were provided in an intensive schedule, 30 hours over four weeks each. The treatments contrasted drill-based vs. communication-based interactions between the client and the clinician. Outcome measures included verb naming and production of personal narratives.
Outcomes & Results: Drill-based but not communication-based treatment had a small positive effect on participants' verb naming accuracy. The communication-based protocol, but not the drill-based treatment, had a pronounced positive effect on participants' sentence and narrative structure.
Conclusions: The results suggest that communication-based interactions are more effective than drill in improving narrative production in aphasia. We suggest that this type of communication-based constraint-induced therapy works to reduce learned non-use patterns of language production and can be structured to improve production of verbs in sentences. The success of this approach can be attributed to the fact communication-based therapy, like typical verbal interactions, emphasises exchange of novel information and allows individuals with aphasia to capitalise on their preserved discourse knowledge.

Keywords: Aphasia; Discourse; Conversation; Therapy; Treatment; Narrative.

Some methods of treating clients with impaired speech and language production associated with aphasia emphasise predominantly drill-based exercises; others emphasise more social, discourse-based client–clinician interactions (Brookshire, 2003; Chapey,

Address correspondence to: Daniel Kempler, Communication Sciences and Disorders, Emerson College, 120 Boylston St., Boston, MA 02116, USA. E-mail: daniel_kempler@emerson.edu

We thank our participants and their families, as well as the following research assistants who participated in collecting and analysing the data: Carmit Altman, Maria Boklan, Caroline Cano, Carol Cayer-Meade, Peggy Conner, Laura Glufling-Tham, Kristen Maul, Youngmi Park, Dagmar Alvarado, Shancia Jarrett, Deepa Sar, Shannon Saul, Vanessa Smith, Tali Swann-Sternberg, Libby Venancio, and Stephanie Wolfe. Support for Mira Goral was provided by NIH grant DC-009792.

http://dx.doi.org/10.1080/02687038.2011.599364

2008; Helm-Estabrooks & Holland, 1998; Hengst, Duff, & Dettmer, 2010; Howard & Hatfield, 1987; Kempler, 2005; Whitworth, Webster, & Howard, 2005).

The "didactic" and "stimulation" methods (Howard & Hatfield, 1987) rely on drill repetition (imitation), phrase and sentence completion, picture naming and, in general, eliciting multiple productions of the target items during each session. These client–clinician interactions do not typically involve exchange of novel information as generally occurs in communication-based verbal interactions in discourse. Hengst et al. (2010) wrote that the use of drill and repetition achieve learning through reinforcement of behaviours and/or "strengthening neuro-pathways that underlie target skills" (p. 888).

In contrast, language can be elicited in treatment in a communicative context, methods sometimes referred to as a "cognitive-contextual", "functional", "sociolinguistic", "communicative", or "pragmatic" (Chapey, 2008; Kempler, 2005). These reflect the fact that language is largely "dialogic" (Hengst et al., 2010) and "transactive" (Wertz, 1998). That is, language is typically used to communicate in a variety of contexts to transfer information between individuals. The verbal interactions are generative or novel in so far as they use words and sentences (as well as gestures, etc.) creatively to communicate information. These aphasia therapy methods generally elicit language production that is relevant, unambiguous and sufficiently informative for that context. The underlying features of these methods are largely adapted from the pragmatically based cooperative principle that guides conversation (Grice, 1975). In order to preserve the pragmatics of conversation these methods may incorporate exchange of novel information between the clients and clinicians in individual dialogues, open-ended group discussions as well as structured barrier tasks.

It should be noted that drill- and communication-based methods are not mutually exclusive and both can be integrated into a single treatment protocol. For instance, script training (e.g., Cherney, Halper, Holland, & Cole, 2008) uses a small number of conversation-based scripts, mastered through repetition. Melodic intonation therapy (Albert, Sparks, & Helm, 1973; Belin et al., 1996) uses a small set of (drill-learned) intonation patterns superimposed on conversational exchanges. The relative preference of any one method might depend on severity of aphasia (more severe symptoms might warrant eliciting speech production through simple sound repetition while milder aphasia might allow for a concentration on discourse structure through novel narrative generation), the goals of the client, the perspective of the clinician, and whether the therapy is provided in an individual or group setting.

Clinical efficacy can be evaluated on the basis of a direct treatment effect such as improved performance on the treated items in the treatment context. However, one of the crucial questions about aphasia therapy is the extent of generalisation achieved by the treatment. Generalisation refers to demonstration of a behavioural response in a different linguistic, interpersonal, or other context not explicitly practised in the treatment. Ideally treatment will result in improvement of untrained lexical items, linguistic structures, communication tasks or settings, and interaction partners.

It is our hypothesis that the type of interaction used in therapy will determine the extent and type of improvement and generalisation found following therapy. We predict that drill-based exercises, because they typically work with a restricted set of items in a non-communicative context, are more likely to result in direct treatment effects, such as improvement on the particular items and tasks practised in therapy. In contrast, we hypothesise that communicative interactions using a less restricted set of practice items are more likely to result in generalisation to a wider array of items and contexts. Greater generalisation in this case might be attributed to the similarity between the therapeutic interactions and other discourse contexts in so far as both incorporate the core discourse principle of information exchange.

While most aphasia treatment research does not explicitly compare drill-based and communication-based treatment methods, recent studies of Constraint Induced Aphasia Therapy (CIAT) have addressed this to some extent. CIAT is built on three principles borrowed from work in Constraint-Induced Movement Therapy with hemiparetic patients (Taub, Uswatte, & Pidikiti, 1999). Based on the notion that brain injury can result in adaptations that substitute easier but non-optimal compensations for lost function (called "learned nonuse"), constraint induced therapy restrains the use of compensatory adaptations (e.g., use of left-hand for patients with right hemiplegia), is intense by emphasising "massed practice" (i.e., movement is often practised all day long), and is functional (i.e., clients engage in real-life activities). These principles have been adapted to aphasia therapy by constraining interaction to verbal channels, implementing relatively intense therapy schedules (massed practice), and using communicative card games such as "Go Fish" to simulate functional communication. Results available to date for the efficacy of CIAT are promising, with participants showing improvement in standardised test measures, direct treatment effects on baseline measures, and generalisation to other contexts by measuring independent ratings of participant communication (Goral & Kempler, 2009; Maher et al., 2006; Pulvermüller et al., 2001). It is not clear from this body of research which aspect(s) of CIAT are most crucial to improved performance. Several studies have demonstrated the importance of constraining therapy to verbal output only, in finding that this type of therapy was more effective than a comparison therapy in which participants could use other modalities as well (Maher et al., 2006; Pulvermüller et al., 2001). However, Barthel and colleagues (Barthel, Meinzer, Djundja, & Rockstroh, 2008) compared two intensive therapies that were communication based, one in which language was limited to verbal output and another in which additional communication modalities were used (e.g., writing). They found that on most measures the two treatments were equally effective. With regard to intensity, there is significant evidence that more intense therapy yields more robust short-term benefits, although the long-term advantage of intense therapy is less clear (Cherney, Patterson, Raymer, Frymark, & Schooling, 2008).

The specific contribution of functionality in CIAT has not been directly addressed. The goal of the present study was to determine the relative importance of functionality in the effectiveness of aphasia therapy. Towards that end we conducted two single-participant studies in which therapy was provided to individuals with moderately severe non-fluent aphasia. Both participants received drill-based and communication-based treatments in sequence to ascertain the relative efficacy of each treatment type on measures of word, sentence and narrative production.

METHOD

Participants

Two women diagnosed with non-fluent aphasia participated in the study. Each had sustained a single left hemisphere thrombo-embolic stroke. Participant #1 (P1) was 54 years old and 2 years post-onset and Participant #2 (P2) was 45 years old and 7 years post onset at the time of treatment. Both participants are right-handed and both demonstrated mild-moderate right hemiparesis. Both participants completed high school and worked prior to their strokes. Following the stroke both received speech-language therapy; neither was engaged in individual therapy other than the experimental treatment reported here for the duration of the study.

The language production of both participants consisted primarily of one-word utterances, few function words, and slow speech production with many pauses. Neither exhibited dysarthria or marked apraxia of speech. Their comprehension skills surpassed their production skills and appeared good in conversational context. At the onset of the study, P1's Western Aphasia Battery (WAB; Kertesz, 1982) aphasia quotient was 75.9 and P2's was 65.2 (see Table 1 later). Neither participant exhibited hearing or visual impairment. The participants volunteered for the study and signed appropriate consent forms.

Treatment protocol

Each participant completed 60 hours of individual treatment. Two different treatment protocols were administered sequentially, each for 30 hours, approximately 7.5 hours per week. Due to their difficulty producing verbs and grammatical sentences, the goal of both treatment protocols was identical: production of appropriate verbs in single sentences. The two protocols differed in the way in which the production was elicited and in what the acceptable targets of production were. Specifically, they differed in two crucial respects: whether the targets were drawn from a finite list of verbs and whether the interactions were communication-based. For the sake of explication, the two protocols are labelled "Drill" and "Generative".

The Drill protocol targeted a set of 32 verbs, selected from the action naming protocol presented in prior work on verb production (Almor et al., 2009) and used in the present study as one of the outcome measures (see outcome measures below for further description of the verb set). An additional set of 32 comparable filler verbs were included in treatment to yield a larger practice set of 64 verbs, but only the 32 targeted items were tested before and after treatment. The Drill protocol provided the participants with highly structured practice of the treated list of verbs. During each session a subset of the target verb list was used in several activities, including sentence repetition, picture description, choral reading, a memory game, and sentence completion. During a given activity, multiple sets of 4–10 spoken or written sentences or picture cards, each depicting an action, were presented to the participant. Prior to each activity the participant rehearsed the items in a three-step process by listening to the clinician's model, repeating the production in unison with the clinician, and then repeating after the clinician's model. Following this rehearsal, the words were practised in the activity. Production was not elicited in a communicative context; rather, in each case, the clinician knew the target and worked through scaffolding to elicit the correct verb and structure. On average each verb was practised approximately 40 times in the course of 30 hours of Drill treatment. Novel pictures depicting the target action verbs were introduced frequently. Therefore there were more than 64 different pictures used to depict the 64 actions/verbs.

In contrast, the Generative protocol did not involve a limited set of preselected verbs. Here the participant was encouraged to generate single sentences containing verbs in grammatical structures to communicate the description of the picture they selected. The Generative protocol relied on verbal games and informative communication-based interactions. Therapy activities included card games, such as Go Fish, a memory game, and a map task, in which the participant and the clinician took turns generating sentences that described actions depicted in picture cards. In these language games all verbal interactions adhered to conversational maxims in that the clinician did not know which card the participant was attempting to describe in a given turn. This was accomplished by use of a physical barrier and duplicate materials. Crucially, in the Generative treatment no clear targets were predetermined; any verb in a sentence, which communicated relevant information, was accepted. The verbs and sentence structures were not rehearsed; modelling was limited to the clinician's productions within the turn taking context of the activities. The emphasis in this therapy was for the participants to develop the habit of generating diverse verbs in sentences in functional contexts, rather than to practice a limited set of preselected verbs. To reinforce the habit of producing verbs, the participant and clinician produced two different but appropriate responses per turn.

Shaping and scaffolding were used throughout both treatments. If the participant did not produce an appropriate verb in a grammatical sentence, the clinician requested the missing information (in the case of omitted verb or other element) and modelled an accurate response as needed. Both participants quickly internalised the rules of the tasks and attempted to produce verbs in sentences in each of their productions. When participants achieved 80% accuracy during in-session probing, the target structure was modified. For example, if a participant was able to produce simple S-V-O structures, the elicited structure was advanced to S-V-O+PP. None of action pictures from the outcome measure was used as stimulus during treatment. See the Appendices for more details of treatment tasks and parameters.

Treatment was provided by student clinicians under direct supervision of the authors. Treatment fidelity was assured by regular discussions to plan and review the protocol and by observation of the sessions.

Pre- and post-testing (outcome measures)

Two measures were administered prior to and following a 3-week period of no treatment (to establish a stable baseline) and before and after each treatment block. One measure assessed verb naming and the other examined narrative production. At each testing time data were collected over three sessions, with a third of the outcome data collected in each of the three sessions. Testing over three sessions allowed us to calculate effect sizes to assess change. A standardised measure, the WAB, was administered once before and after each treatment block.

Verb naming. A set of 96 action pictures was used to elicit verb naming in sentences (Almor et al., 2009). All of the verbs were highly imageable, familiar, and with high (87%) overall naming agreement. The verbs were divided into three comparable lists; one list was treated during the Drill protocol. The outcome measure for the verb-naming task was the number of target verbs accurately produced. We counted as correct only those verbs that were expected as targets in the Almor study (e.g., for a picture of a girl "balancing" on a beam, the verb "practising", although describing the picture, was not counted as correct). Verbs that are homophones of nouns (e.g., to iron/an iron) were only counted as verbs if there was evidence in the sentence to support this (e.g., in a picture of a woman ironing a shirt, a single word production "iron" was not counted as a verb; the production of "iron" in: "the woman iron the shirt" was). For Drill treatment we examined naming accuracy for treated and untreated items.

Narrative production. Three personal narratives (a vacation; a happy moment for you or someone in your family; and a movie, book, or TV show that you enjoyed) were elicited prior to and following each treatment block. Narratives were elicited with a minimum of prompting. The participants were prompted to tell a different narrative each time so they did not tell the story of the same vacation, happy moment, or movie on each testing. The recorded narratives were transcribed, checked by another investigator, and divided into utterances. To identify each utterance, we modified Foster, Tonkyn, and Wigglesworth's (2000, p. 366) notion of an Analysis of Speech Unit (AS-Unit), defined as any independent clause (that minimally includes a finite verb) as well as any sub-clausal unit, "which can be elaborated to a full clause by means of recovery of ellipted elements from the context of the discourse . . .". Identifying each individual AS-Unit took into consideration intonation contour, pauses, meaning, and syntactic construction. We modified the original definition to apply to utterances as minimal as a single word, even in instances when the missing elements were difficult to infer from the context.

The outcome measures for the narratives included lexical, sentence, and discourse variables as follows. Because treatment focused on verb production, our lexical measures were Total verbs (the total number of verbs produced), Verb diversity (the number of different verb types), and Verb form (the number of correctly conjugated verb forms). The sentence-level variables included the Lexical density of utterances (proportion of content words of total words) as well as whether or not the utterances were complete and grammatical. Utterance completeness was rated using the AS-Unit scale described above, taking into account both the complexity of the structure and presence of obligatory elements. Note that utterances could be complete if they contained all the obligatory elements even if the end result was not grammatical due to poor grammatical form (e.g., "The birds is eating the kitten"). To determine sentence completeness, AS-Units were identified and then rated on a 5-point scale: 1 = incomplete sentence; 2 = simple and complete, containing all obligatory elements; 3 = complex sentence containing an incomplete subordinate clause; 4 = complete coordinate structure; 5 = complete containing a subordinate structure. Grammatical utterances contained all obligatory elements and adhered to grammatical rules of English.

Discourse variables included two measures of productivity: Total number of words (not including exact repetitions, false starts, interjections, or formulaic expressions) and Total number of utterances; and three measures of narrative structure: Local coherence, Global coherence, and Story line ratio. Local coherence was gauged by whether each utterance was directly related to the prior utterance by elaboration, sequencing, focus, etc. Global coherence refers to the relevance of each utterance to the general topic. For the coherence measures we used a 3-point scale (1 = unrelated, 2 = possibly related, and 3 = clearly related), modified from Coelho and Flewellyn (2003). The final discourse measure, Story line ratio, was the number of utterances that described a clear story line divided by the number of utterances that contained a description of the setting or background for the narrative (Longacre, as reported by Olness, 2006). The WAB subtests related to spontaneous speech, auditory-verbal comprehension, repetition and word finding were administered before and after each treatment block and an aphasia quotient was calculated.

ANALYSIS AND RESULTS

All testing sessions were recorded and transcribed for later analysis. The transcripts were coded for variables of interest by individuals blind to treatment conditions. Approximately 20% of each transcript was re-coded by a second individual, with inter-rater reliability ranging between 93% and 99% for each transcript; disagreements were resolved by discussion with the authors. In the results that follow we evaluated change using effect sizes based on means and standard deviations of results from the three testing sessions prior to and following each treatment. Effect sizes were calculated by subtracting the pre-treatment mean from the post-treatment mean, divided by the pre-treatment standard deviation. Although there has been debate about how to determine whether an effect size represents a meaningful change (e.g., Beeson & Robey, 2006; Robey, 1998), we follow Raymer and colleagues (e.g., Raymer et al., 2007; Rodriguez, Raymer, & Gonzalez Rothi, 2006) in interpreting as clinically significant improvement a positive effect size greater than 2.5 with a change of greater than 20% from baseline. Three of the narrative variables reported below (Sentence completeness, Local and Global coherence) were measured on a limited nominal scale. For these, pre- to post-treatment change was assessed using non-parametric Mann–Whitney comparisons based on all items across the three testing sessions before and following each treatment rather than means of each testing session, due to the lack of variability inherent in the measure and brevity of some of the narratives. For these variables, we used an alpha level of .05. We report below the results for the standardised testing and our two experimental tasks: Verb naming and Narrative production.

Standardised testing

Performance on the WAB showed minimal increase following each treatment type (see Table 1). The extent of change did not exceed five points and therefore is not considered clinically significant (Katz & Wertz, 1997).

Verb naming

The results of the verb naming are presented in Table 2. Overall, mean naming accuracy for the 96 items did not change significantly for either participant following

TABLE 1
Western Aphasia Battery (WAB) results

	Drill		*Generative*	
P1	*Pre*	*Post*	*Pre*	*Post*
Spontaneous speech	14	15	14	15
Auditory verbal comprehension	7.3	7.9	8.3	8.6
Repetition	8.1	7.6	6.6	6.8
Naming & word finding	8	8.8	8.5	8.6
Aphasia Quotient	74.8	78.6	74.8	78
	Drill		*Generative*	
P2	*Pre*	*Post*	*Pre*	*Post*
Spontaneous speech	11	12	12	14
Auditory verbal comprehension	10	9.95	9.95	10
Repetition	5.1	4.4	4.4	4.2
Naming & word finding	7.8	8.5	8.2	8.2
Aphasia Quotient	67.8	69.7	69.1	72.8

TABLE 2
Verb naming results

P1	Drill: # items named correctly before tx	Drill: # items named correctly after tx	Drill: # items named correctly after tx that were not named before tx	Generative: # items named correctly before tx	Generative: # items named correctly after tx
All ($n = 96$)	55	66	12	65	57
Treated ($n = 32$)	18	21	3	n/a	n/a
Untreated ($n = 64$)	37	45	9	n/a	n/a
P2					
All ($n = 96$)	63	67	18	68	69
Treated ($n = 32$)	18	28	11	n/a	n/a
Untreated ($n = 64$)	45	39	7	n/a	n/a

either treatment (P1: pre-treatment $M = 18.3$, $SD = 2.5$; post-treatment $M = 22.0$, $SD = 2.6$; effect size = 1.5; P2: pre-treatment $M = 21.0$, $SD = 7.9$; post-treatment $M = 22.3$, $SD = 7.4$; effect size = .17). When we examined the change in the 32 treated items before vs after Drill treatment, we observed a numerical increase in number of correctly produced verbs for both participants (from 18 to 21 for P1 and from 18 to 28 for P2). This increase can be taken as direct treatment effect: following Drill treatment P1 named all the verbs she had named prior to the treatment plus three additional verbs she had not named accurately before; P2 named all the verbs she had named before Drill treatment except one and named 11 additional verbs that she had not named before the treatment. Those 11 verbs were practised on average during treatment as often as other verbs among the 32 trained items. On the 64 untreated items, the two participants had different patterns: P1 increased naming accuracy (from 37 to 45) while P2 decreased in naming accuracy (from 45 to 39).

Following Generative treatment there was no improvement in total accuracy (P1 decreased in total accuracy from 65 to 57; P2 named 68 correct verbs pre and 69 post Generative treatment). In the Generative treatment no verbs were targeted for treatment so a comparison of treated vs untreated items is not applicable. Nor was there change when the test was administered following a period of no treatment (P1: Pre $M = 18.0$, $SD = 0$; Post $M = 18.0$, $SD = 2.6$; effect size not calculable due to pre-treatment SD of 0; P2: Pre $M = 12.7$, $SD = 2.9$; Post $M = 14.0$, $SD = 3.0$; effect size = .46).

Narrative production

We report below the results for variables at the lexical, sentence, and discourse levels derived from the narrative production. Overall, the participants produced better narratives after Generative but not Drill treatment. The narrative results are presented in Tables 3 and 4.

TABLE 3
Comparison of narrative outcomes following Drill and Generative treatments for P1

P1	Drill treatment			Generative treatment		
	Pre Mean (SD)	*Post Mean (SD)*	*Effect size (ES) or Mann–Whitney (p)*	*Pre Mean (SD)*	*Post Mean (SD)*	*Effect size (ES) or Mann–Whitney (p)*
			Lexical variables			
Total verbs	6.0 (0)	4.67 (3.79)	NA	7.33 (2.52)	13.33 (2.21)	ES = 2.38*
Verb diversity	4.67 (1.53)	3.33 (3.21)	ES < 1	5 (2.0)	9.00 (3.46)	ES = 2.00*
Verb form	3.67 (2.52)	4.33 (3.21)	ES < 1	6.33 (3.21)	9.67 (4.04)	ES = 1.04*
			Sentence variables			
Lexical density	0.65 (.01)	0.55 (.30)	ES–7.29	0.41 (.07)	0.51 (.03)	ES = 1.50
Sentence completeness	1.85 (.12)	1.83 (.15)	P > .1	1.48 (.16)	1.77 (.39)	**p = .03***
Grammatical utterances	2.67 (2.08)	3.00 (1.73)	ES < 1	3.33 (.58)	6.33 (2.89)	**ES = 5.20***
			Discourse variables			
Total words	24.67 (2.89)	16.67 (12.90)	ES = −2.77	37 (16.52)	48 (11.36)	ES < 1
Total utterances	6.33 (1.53)	5.67 (4.04)	ES < 1	10.67 (4.16)	12.33 (3.06)	ES < 1
Local coherence	2.26 (.05)	2.45 (.48)	p = .066	1.89 (.62)	2.44 (.36)	**p < .001***
Global coherence	2.58 (.52)	2.18 (1.02)	p = .075	2.49 (.46)	2.86 (.07)	**p = .001***
Story line ratio	2.22 (2.41)	.22 (.38)	ES < 1	0.47 (.46)	3.21 (4.16)	**ES = 5.95***

NA = Effect size could not be calculated due to a pre-treatment standard deviation of 0; * = improvement of more than 20% but effect size < 2.5; * & **bold** = effect size greater than 2.5 and > 20% improvement or $p < .05$ (Mann–Whitney).

TABLE 4
Comparison of narrative outcomes following Drill and Generative treatments for P2

P2	Drill treatment			Generative treatment		
	Pre Mean (SD)	*Post Mean (SD)*	*Effect size (ES) or Mann–Whitney (p)*	*Pre Mean (SD)*	*Post Mean (SD)*	*Effect size (ES) or Mann–Whitney (p)*
Lexical variables						
Total verbs	1 (1.73)	0 (0)	ES < 1	1.67 (1.12)	5.0 (2.0)	**ES = 2.89***
Verb diversity	1 (1.73)	0 (0)	ES < 1	0.67 (.58)	5.0 (2.0)	**ES = 7.51***
Verb form	.33 (.58)	0 (0)	ES < 1	0.33 (.58)	2.67 (3.06)	**ES = 4.04***
Sentence variables						
Lexical density	0.39 (.05)	.40 (.04)	ES < 1	0.52 (.22)	.44 (.05)	ES < 1
Sentence completeness	1 (0)	1 (0)	p > .1	1 (0)	1.67 (.23)	**p = .002***
Grammatical utterances	0.33 (.58)	0 (0)	ES < 1	0 (0)	1.67 (1, 53)	NA
Discourse variables						
Total words	9 (5.57)	6.33 (1.53)	ES < 1	10.33 (2.08)	37.33 (12.58)	**ES = 12.97***
Total utterances	3.33 (1.53)	2.67 (1.15)	ES < 1	2.33 (1.53)	7.33 (.58)	**ES = 3.27**
Local coherence	2.33 (.58)	2.00 (0)	p > .1	1.44 (1.26)	2.89 (.19)	**p = .049***
Global coherence	2.5 (.50)	2.67 (.58)	P > .1	1.44 (1.26)	2.89 (.19)	**p = .049***
Story line ratio	0.5 (.87)	0 (0)	ES < 1	0.17 (.29)	3.39 (3.26)	**ES = 11.16***

NA = Effect size could not be calculated due to a pre-treatment standard deviation of 0; * = improvement of more than 20% but effect size < 2.5; * & **bold** = effect size greater than 2.5 and > 20% improvement or $p < .05$ (Mann–Whitney).

Lexical variables

The narratives of both participants contained a greater number of verbs, greater range of verbs (verb diversity), and more accurate verb form following Generative but not Drill treatment. Specifically, the lexical measures showed positive albeit modest effect for P1 (increase of 20% from baseline on all three measures but effect sizes smaller than 2.5) and medium-to-large effect sizes (between 2.89 and 7.5 with increases of at least 20%) on all three measures for P2.

Sentence variables

Overall, sentence quality improved following Generative but not Drill treatment. Both participants produced a significantly greater number of complete utterances (see sentence completeness in Tables 3 and 4) and more grammatical utterances following Generative treatment. P1 produced a greater number of grammatical utterances following Generative treatment (effect size = 5.2) despite the fact that she did not produce more utterances overall following either treatment. P2 also produced more grammatical utterances following Generative treatment, but an effect size could not be calculated because she produced no grammatical utterances prior to Generative treatment (a pre-treatment SD of 0 cannot be used to calculate an effect size). The only sentence-level measure that showed no positive change for either participant following either treatment was Lexical density (i.e., proportion of content words compared to all words) within utterances.

Discourse variables

The discourse measures overall showed improvement following Generative but not Drill treatment. On the measures of overall narrative productivity—the number of words and utterances each participant produced before and after treatment—P1 did not change following either treatment; P2 produced substantially longer narratives following Generative (but not Drill) treatment. All three measures of internal narrative structure changed towards typical values following Generative but not Drill treatment. Specifically, both participants produced more utterances that clearly related to the overall narrative topic (Global coherence) and more utterances related to immediately preceding utterances (Local coherence) after Generative treatment. Moreover, the post-Generative narratives contained more utterances relating punctiliar events (story-line elements) that were judged to move the narrative forward than the pre-Generative narratives. The same was not seen comparing performance prior to and following Drill treatment.

SUMMARY AND DISCUSSION

Two women with chronic non-fluent aphasia participated in language treatment designed to improve verb production in sentences. Each participant received two treatment protocols, provided in sequence. The two protocols contrasted drill-based vs communication-based interactions between the participant and the clinician. Outcome measures, administered before and after each treatment block, examined the production of verbs in an action picture description task and production of personal narratives. Drill treatment, which relied on repetition, had a positive albeit small effect on participants' verb naming accuracy. The Generative treatment had a pronounced positive effect on participants' use of verbs in self-generated narratives as well as on their sentence and narrative structure.

Aphasiologists acknowledge that many treatment approaches in aphasia can bring about change in language behaviours that are directly related to those addressed in treatment. However, a more challenging task has been to demonstrate consistent generalisation from language produced during treatment to language use outside treatment (e.g., Edmonds, Nadeau, & Kiran, 2009; Links, Hurkmans, & Bastiaanse, 2010; Peach & Reuter, 2010; Rose & Sussmilch, 2008).

In the present study improved verb naming for items that were practised during treatment would be evidence of a direct treatment effect, whereas increased naming accuracy for verbs that were not practised in therapy would be considered generalisation to untreated items; improvement on narrative production would be taken as generalisation to an untrained task. One of our participants (P2) demonstrated a direct treatment effect following Drill therapy, as her naming accuracy increased on treated items. She showed little evidence of generalisation to untreated items. This is similar to other studies that have reported a lack of generalisation to unpractised verbs following various verb-training protocols (e.g., Raymer et al., 2007; Webster, Morris, & Franklin, 2005). The other participant (P1) showed evidence of improvement on verb naming overall, as she named more treated and untreated items following Drill treatment. We conclude that, overall, the verb-naming measure demonstrated generally positive outcomes. That is, practising the production of specific verbs during treatment led to increased ability to produce these verbs and, to some degree, to increased ability to produce other verbs in a task similar to one used during treatment. As may be expected, neither participant named more target verbs in the action description task following the Generative treatment, as the participants did not directly practise any of the verbs used in the outcome measure during this treatment. However, following Generative treatment both participants improved their verb production in narratives.

One of our primary questions was whether treatment improved language production that is more typical of language use outside therapy. To gauge general language use we analysed personal narratives that the participants produced before and after each treatment. This measure differed from the treatment tasks, in that telling personal narratives required participants to generate multiple linked utterances without visual support of pictures. Personal narratives are an appropriate assessment of functional language use as they occur in many discourse contexts from reporting daily events to telling jokes and stories, and can contribute to an individual's ability to understand life experiences, present oneself to others, and participate in various communal and communicative events. Indeed, it might be argued that one ultimate goal of aphasia treatment is functional production and comprehension of narratives.

The results of our narrative analyses were consistent and striking: The only marked changes in these measures for either participant were seen after Generative but not Drill treatment. While there were some differences in the strength of findings for the two participants, they both showed improvements on measures of lexical diversity, sentence structure, and discourse in their narratives following Generative but not the Drill treatment. These results are discussed below in the context of other similar findings in the literature.

First, our findings of greater verb diversity and more accurate verb forms in narratives following Generative treatment are consistent with a recent study reporting treatment generalisation to elicited connected speech (Links et al., 2010). Links and colleagues trained verb and sentence production using a program they developed and termed ACTION, in which verbs are elicited at four levels (single verbs, filling in infinitives, filling in finite verbs, and sentence construction). They examined a number of variables to assess change in discourse production following treatment and reported positive change for some of their participants on two lexical measures comparable to ours, namely those pertaining to verb diversity and verb morphology. They also found, similar to the improvement we documented for sentence completeness for our participants, that 9 of their 11 participants produced longer sentences following treatment.

Second, the improvement in sentence structure we documented (more complete and more grammatically correct utterances) reflects a better ability to retrieve the required elements of the sentence, and is similar to the generalisation findings reported in two recent studies. Edmonds et al. (2009) trained the production of verbs in conjunction with thematic roles and then used a picture description task to elicit connected speech to examine treatment generalisation. They found that, following treatment, their participants produced both the subject and the verb in the sentence more often than prior to treatment, and that three of their four participants produced more complete utterances following treatment. Similarly, Webster et al. (2005) treated one person's verb production deficit using activities that required verb production, noun–verb association, and sentence generation, and demonstrated that their participant produced a greater variety of argument structures and omitted fewer obligatory items in connected speech following treatment.

Finally, to our knowledge, discourse structure has not been examined in prior studies of verb therapy in aphasia. Our results showing impaired narrative coherence prior to treatment support Coehlo and Flewellyn's (2003) finding that macrolinguistic abilities are impaired in aphasia; our findings of improved discourse coherence following treatment suggest that therapy incorporating basic discourse principles can be helpful in improving these elements of narrative production.

Why was Generative treatment more effective than Drill treatment for improving narrative production? In order to address this question we discuss here how the two treatments were similar and how they differed. Both treatments were similar in so far as they adhered to two principles familiar from descriptions of Constraint Induced Aphasia Therapy (CIAT): massed practice and constrained language use (Goral & Kempler, 2009; Maher et al., 2006; Pulvermüller et al., 2001). Massed practice was implemented by administering both treatments with a relatively intense schedule of 7.5 hours a week for 4 weeks. Constraint was implemented in both therapies by emphasising the use of verbal modality and the expected use of verbs in every sentence. The therapeutic use of only spoken language and frequent verb production were motivated by the theory of learned non-use in which a less-impaired skill becomes a new standard as an individual with a brain injury learns to avoid a relatively impaired function and rely on a relatively spared function (Lillie & Mateer, 2006; Pulvermüller et al., 2001; Taub, Uswatte, Mark, & Morris, 2006). From this perspective, persons with aphasia come to rely on non-verbal communication modalities and, if they produce verbal language, they rely on those language components that are most easily accessible to them. For individuals with non-fluent, agrammatic aphasia, this means they often rely on the production of nouns in verbal communication rather than struggle to produce complete sentences containing verbs. The sole use of the verbal modality was exercised here to avoid compensatory use of less-impaired communication modalities, such as gesture and drawing; the requirement for production of verbs was motivated to reduce an over-reliance on nouns. Since both treatments required participants to produce a spoken verb on every turn despite their difficulty in doing so, the simple act of producing verbs cannot explain the different outcomes of the two treatment protocols.

The two treatments diverged with regard to a third principle of CIAT—the one we set out to examine in the present study—functionality. Specifically, the tasks used in the two treatments differ in whether or not they were designed to communicate new information. The Drill treatment relies on the clinician modelling target responses and the participant repeating, reading aloud, describing action pictures, and participating in choral reading. Therefore the Drill therapy does not involve exchange of new information. In contrast, in the Generative treatment there are no target responses modelled by the clinician and the language productions are relatively unscripted. On each turn, there are a variety of possible and acceptable responses. Each turn is designed to transmit relatively novel information, capitalising on preserved pragmatics of cooperative discourse such as turn taking and maintaining contextual relevance, in structured language tasks designed to elicit single sentences. These elements are neither relevant nor called into use during Drill therapy and are, in fact, artificially suspended for the drill-based exercises. We suggest that integrating the discourse principle of informative exchanges into Generative therapy enhanced the generalisation of the practised tasks (production of verbs in single sentences describing action pictures) to another discourse context (production of self-generated narratives consisting of linked utterances without the visual support of pictures).

The integration of novel information exchange in the Generative treatment makes it similar to therapeutic approaches that emphasise the importance of conversational context, such as Supported Conversation and the Life Participation Approach to Aphasia (e.g., Kagan, Black, Duchan, Simmons-Mackie, & Square, 2001; Kagan et al., 2008; Simmons-Mackie, 2008). These approaches emphasise the social-functional context of aphasia and aim to bridge the disparity that often exists between gains that people with aphasia achieve in treatment sessions vs. their ability to carry over these improvements to other communicative and discourse contexts.

Generative therapy is similar to conversation-based treatments in so far as they both are based on the communication of novel information. However, unlike conversational treatment contexts, (1) our tasks constrained participant responses to verbal productions only (as opposed to encouraging the use a wide array of communication modalities) and (2) required participants to generate single sentences, neither connected to one another nor to a unifying thematic context. This structure allowed us to address our participants' specific deficits and focus on restoring the habit of producing spoken sentences containing verbs. We postulate that the combination of focusing on the use of verbs in spoken language production and communicative exchanges helped the participants to begin undoing the learned non-use of verbs in sentences.

Another reason Generative treatment might be more likely to generalise is that it required participants to self-generate sentences, which is similar to most other communicative activities including our narrative outcome measures. This is not true of Drill therapy in which responses were modelled for the participant. We note that many of the verbs the participants produced in their post-Generative narratives were not produced more than a few times in the course of the 30 hours of treatment. Of the 14 verbs produced by P2 in the post-Generative narratives, 10 were produced during the therapy sessions fewer than 10 times each and only 3 were practised more than 15 times; similarly, half of the verbs produced by P1 in her post-Generative narratives were used during treatment 10 times or fewer. Therefore it was not the production of specific verbs that improved following Generative treatment but the ability to use verbs more consistently during language production.

Finally, another advantage of the Generative treatment might be the fact that it is more engaging and motivating than the Drill approach simply because the information exchange is more typical of daily language use. Integrating this discourse principle into the therapy technique allows participants to use their intact conversational and pragmatic skills. Whereas we do not deny the value of some drill-based practice in aphasia treatment, we take our results as evidence for a limited carryover afforded by repeated practice of specific items in a non-communicative context.

The results of this study should be interpreted carefully given several limitations. First, the findings should be replicated with additional participants before we can generalise these findings to a wider population. Second, the two treatments we employed were administered sequentially—both of our participants received Drill treatment prior to Generative treatment. Therefore it is possible that the Generative treatment was more effective in improving narrative production simply because it was the second treatment, and the improvement is due to a cumulative effect of hours of treatment, not the type of treatment. We do not believe this to be the case for several reasons: Our participants were both individuals with chronic aphasia, well past a period of spontaneous improvement, who had shown only modest gains in traditional therapy before this study, and made no progress on our outcome measures during a 3-week period of no treatment prior to this study, nor during the intense course of Drill treatment. Therefore we think it is reasonable to attribute the improvements we observed to the properties of the Generative therapy protocol. Similarly, it is possible that improvement on the outcomes measures after the second treatment was due to a practice effect associated with the repeated administration of these measures. However, this appears unlikely as we elicited different specific narratives (i.e., different vacations, different movies) at each testing time, making it unlikely that the participants had merely gotten better at telling a particular story. Also of note, two other data points from our laboratory, not reported here, support these conclusions: (1) a prior published study with a comparable (i.e., chronic, non-fluent) participant demonstrated that Generative treatment elicited significant positive results (Goral & Kempler, 2009) while a drill-based treatment with the same individual following the Generative treatment did not show continued gains; (2) one of the participants in the study reported here (P2) received additional non-generative treatment following the Generative treatment reported here, and did not demonstrate additional functional language gains. Nonetheless we recommend that future work counterbalance the order of treatments to study a potential contribution of treatment order to the effects reported here.

Another question unanswered by this research is whether the effectiveness of Generative therapy depends on the severity and/or language profile of the person with aphasia. Our participants were similar in that they were relatively young and demonstrated chronic, moderate non-fluent symptoms. Despite these similarities, their language production and responses to treatment differed to a degree. P2, who produced shorter and fewer spontaneous utterances with fewer verbs than P1 at the start of the study, showed greater improvement than P1 at the lexical level after Generative treatment. By contrast, P1 included verbs in many of her utterances prior to treatment and her main improvement was characterised by significant changes at the sentence and discourse levels. Therefore it appears that this type of protocol, which can be adjusted to target output of various levels of utterance complexity (verb alone, SVO, SVO+PP), can have a positive effect for participants with a range of verbal output levels. Both our participants were ideal for this research protocol because, while their spontaneous speech was severely limited, they had the residual ability to produce target items and structures in a structured context with a minimum of scaffolding. However, it remains to be seen if the efficacy of the Generative treatment is comparable for participants with more or less severe as well as different symptoms.

Finally, we used only one outcome measure of connected language use (personal narratives). We acknowledge that story telling is only one aspect of typical language use and may not be representative of performance in conversation and other ways in which people use language to communicate. Future research will be strengthened by including a wider range of outcome measures, to assess other aspects of functional language, including measures of social validation of treatment-related change.

REFERENCES

Albert, M. L., Sparks, R. W., & Helm, N. A. (1973). Melodic intonation therapy for aphasia. *Archives of Neurology, 29*, 130–131.

Almor, A., Aronoff, J. M., MacDonald, M. C., Gonnerman, L. M., Kempler, D., Hintiryan, H., et al. (2009). A common mechanism in verb and noun naming deficits in Alzheimer's patients. *Brain and Language, 111*(1), 8–19.

Barthel, G., Meinzer, M., Djundja, D., & Rockstroh, B. (2008). Intensive language therapy in chronic aphasia: Which aspects contribute most? *Aphasiology, 22*, 408–421.

Beeson, P. M., & Robey, R. (2006). Evaluating single-subject treatment research: Lessons learned from the aphasia literature. *Neuropsychological Review, 16*, 161–169.

Belin, P., Van Eeckhout, Ph., Zilbovicius, M., Remy, Ph., Francois, C., Guillaume, S., et al. (1996). Recovery from nonfluent aphasia after melodic intonation therapy. *Neurology, 47*, 1504, 1511.

Brookshire, R. H. (2003). *Introduction to neurogenic communication disorders*. St. Louis, MO: Mosby.

Chapey, R. (2008). *Language intervention strategies in aphasia and related neurogenic communication disorders* (5th ed.). Philadelphia, PA: Wolter Kluwers/Lippincott, Williams & Wilkins.

Cherney, L. R., Halper, A. S., Holland, A. L., & Cole, R. (2008). Computerized script training for aphasia: Preliminary results. *American Journal of Speech-Language Pathology, 17*, 19–34.

Cherney, L. R., Patterson, J. P., Raymer, A., Frymark, T., & Schooling, T. (2008). Evidence-based systematic review: Effect of intensity of treatment and constraint-induced language therapy for individuals with stroke-induced aphasia. *Journal of Speech, Language and Hearing Research, 51*, 1282–1299.

Coelho, C. A., & Flewellyn, L. (2003). Longitudinal assessment of coherence in an adult with fluent aphasia: A follow-up study. *Aphasiology, 17*(2), 173–182.

Edmonds, L. A., Nadeau, S. E., & Kiran, S. (2009). Effect of verb network strengthening treatment (VNeST) on lexical retrieval of content words in sentences in persons with aphasia. *Aphasiology, 23*, 402–424.

Foster, P., Tonkyn, A., & Wigglesworth, G. (2000). Measuring spoken language: A unit for all reasons. *Applied Linguistics, 21*(3), 354–375.

Goral, M., & Kempler, D. (2009). Training verb production in communicative context: Evidence from a person with chronic non-fluent aphasia. *Aphasiology, 23*(12), 1383–1397

Grice, H. P. (1975). Logic and conversation. In P. Cole & J. L. Morgan (Eds.), *Speech acts, syntax and semantics* (Vol. 3, pp. 41–58). New York, NY: Academic Press.

Helm-Estabrooks, N., & Holland, A. (1998). *Approaches to the treatment of aphasia*. San Diego: Singular.

Hengst, J. A., Duff, M. D, & Dettmer, A. (2010). Rethinking repetition in therapy: Repeated engagement as the social ground of learning. *Aphasiology, 24*, 887–901.

Howard, D., & Hatfied, F. M. (1987). *Aphasia therapy: Historical and contemporary issues*. Hove, UK: Lawrence Erlbaum Associates.

Kagan, A., Black, S. E., Duchan, J. F., Simmons-Mackie, N., & Square, P. (2001). Training volunteers as conversation partners using 'Supported Conversation for Adults with Aphasia' (SCA): A controlled trial. *Journal of Speech, Language and Hearing Research, 44*, 624–638.

Kagan, A., Simmons-Mackie, N., Rowland, A., Huijbregts, M., Shumway, E., McEwen, S., et al. (2008) Counting what counts: A framework for capturing real-life outcomes of aphasia intervention. *Aphasiology, 22*(3), 258–280.

Katz, R., & Wertz, R. T. (1997). The efficacy of computer provided reading treatment for chronic aphasic adults. *Journal of Speech, Language, and Hearing Research, 40*, 493–507.

Kempler, D. (2005). *Neurocognitive disorders in aging*. Thousand Oaks, CA: Sage Publications.

Kertesz, A. (1982). *Western Aphasia Battery*. New York, NY: Grune & Stratton.

Lillie, R., & Mateer, C. A. (2006). Constraint-based therapies as a proposed model for cognitive rehabilitation. *Journal of Head Trauma Rehabilitation, 21*(2), 119–130.

Links, P., Hurkmans, J., & Bastiaanse, R. (2010). Training verb and sentence production in agrammatic Broca's aphasia. *Aphasiology, 24*(11), 1303–1325.

Maher, L. M., Kendall, D., Swearengin, J. A., Rodriquez, A., Leon, S. A., Pingel, K., et al. (2006). A pilot study of use-dependent learning in the context of constraint induced language therapy. *Journal of the International Neuropsychological Society, 12*, 843–852.

Olness, G. S. (2006). Genre, verb, and coherence in picture-elicited discourse of adults with aphasia. *Aphasiology, 20*, 175–187

Peach, R., & Reuter, K. (2010). A discourse-based approach to semantic feature analysis for the treatment of aphasic word retrieval failures. *Aphasiology, 24*, 971–990.

Pulvermüller, F., Neininger, B., Elbert, T., Mohr, B., Rockstroh, B., Koebbel, P., et al. (2001). Constraint-induced therapy of chronic aphasia after stroke. *Stroke, 32*, 1621–1626.

Raymer, A. M., Ciampitti, M., Holliway, B., Singletary, F., Blonder, L. X., Ketterson, T., et al. (2007). Semantic-phonologic treatment for noun and verb retrieval impairments in aphasia. *Neuropsychological Rehabilitation, 17*, 244–270.

Robey, R. R. (1998). A meta-analysis of clinical outcomes in the treatment of aphasia. *Journal of Speech, Language, and Hearing Research, 41*(1), 172–187.

Rodriguez, A. D., Raymer, A. M., & Gonzalez Rothi, L. J. (2006). Effects of gesture+verbal and semantic-phonologic treatments for verb retrieval in aphasia. *Aphasiology, 20*, 286–297.

Rose, M., & Sussmilch, G. (2008). The effects of semantic and gesture treatment on verb retrieval and verb use in aphasia. *Aphasiology, 22*, 691–706.

Simmons-Mackie, N. (2008). Social approaches to aphasia intervention. In R. Chapey (Ed.), *Language intervention strategies in aphasia and related neurogenic communication disorders* (pp. 290–318). New York, NY: Lippincott, Williams & Wilkins.

Taub, E., Uswatte, G., Mark, V. W., & Morris, D. M. (2006). The learned nonuse phenomenon: Implications for rehabilitation. *Europa Medicophysica, 42*(3), 241–256.

Taub, E., Uswatte, G., & Pidikiti, R. (1999). Constraint-induced movement therapy: A new family of techniques with broad application to physical rehabilitation – a clinical review. *Journal of Rehabilitation Research and Development, 36*(3), 237–251.

Webster, J., Morris, J., & Franklin, S. (2005). Effects of therapy targeted at verb retrieval and the realization of the predicate argument structure: A case study. *Aphasiology, 19*, 748–764.

Wertz, R. T. (1998). A case of aphasia, apraxia of speech, and apraxia of phonation. In N. Helm-Estabrooks & A. Holland (Eds.), *Approaches to the treatment of aphasia* (pp. 25–38). San Diego, CA: Singular Publishing Group.

Whitworth, A., Webster, J., & Howard, D. (2005). *A cognitive neuropsychological approach to assessment and intervention in aphasia*. New York, NY: Psychology Press.

APPENDIX A

	Drill protocol	*Generative protocol*
Target responses	Both Drill and Generative treatment required spoken production of well-formed sentences containing verbs.	
Guiding principles	Elicitation of target items and structures through repetition with maximum support of auditory modelling and visual stimuli. No new information is exchanged; all production targets are predetermined. Both clinician and participant know the target for each production.	Production of appropriate verbs in sentences in communicative exchanges. Each production was spontaneously produced in language games without a direct model. The clinician and the participant did not have shared knowledge of the precise target in each turn.
Target verbs	A set of 64 verbs was used for the duration of the treatment. From the action naming outcome measure 32 verbs were selected. The additional 32 were added to increase the practice pool. Productions of target verbs were elicited by auditory models, written stimuli, and action pictures. All verbs were concrete and picturable. Both transitive and intransitive verbs were included to accommodate various sentence structures (see "shaping" below).	No set of target verbs was predetermined. Any verb appropriate for the treatment activity was considered correct. Moreover, more than one verb would be considered a correct "target" for a particular action if the verb was appropriate and sufficient to distinguish that action from others (e.g., both "sit" and "wait" may be appropriate to describe a picture of a person sitting at a bus stop as long as both verbs distinguished that picture from others in an array). Productions were elicited by using a wide variety of pictures containing one or more actions in the tasks described below.
Target sentence structures	In both Drill and Generative treatment, target sentence structure varied with participant ability and was shaped throughout therapy. The goal was always for the participant to produce a verb in a well-formed sentence that was difficult but not impossible for the participant to produce. The target sentence structure had the potential to develop through the course of the therapy from an isolated verb in the present progressive form (e.g., "writing") to an SV(O)+PP sentence structure (e.g., "The, man is writing a letter at the desk.") (see "Shaping" below for intermediate steps between these two structures).	
Scaffolding	Three levels of scaffolding were used in all tasks: (1) general prompt, (2) more specific prompt, and (3) a model for repetition. For example in a picture description task in Drill therapy focused on SVO structure, if the participant omitted the verb from a sentence, the general prompt would be "Could you say that sentence with a verb?"; If not successful, the more specific would be "What is the person doing?"; if still not successful, the correct response would be modelled and the participant would be asked to repeat. After two unsuccessful attempts at repetition, the clinician moved on to the next item. The precise prompts were tailored to specific activity and target structure.	
Shaping	Shaping was aimed at increasing the length and complexity of the sentence structures produced by the participants. The target sentence structures had the potential to progress though the following sequence: present progressive verb in isolation ("ironing") > S-V ("The man is yelling") > S-V-O ("The lady is tossing the salad.") > S-V-O-PP ("The boy is rowing a boat in a river."). We targeted one structure at a time. The participant advanced to the next more complex target structure when each structure was mastered (performed the task with 80% or greater accuracy). Accuracy was monitored by probing the client's production of the verbs within the target structure every 3 to 6 hours of treatment (or approximately 5–10 times during the course of each 4-week treatment protocol).	

APPENDIX B

Treatment tasks

Drill protocol

Prior to each activity, the participant rehearsed the target items in a three-step process by listening to the clinician's model, repeating the production in unison with the clinician, and then repeating after the clinician's model. Following this rehearsal, the target items were practised in the activities below.

Verb/Sentence repetition
The clinician produces a target response for a particular picture stimulus, the participant repeats the target.

Picture description
The participant turns over one picture card at a time and describes it with the (prerehearsed) sentence.

Map task
The participant and the clinician view a single sheet of paper with multiple actions pictures displayed in a random spatial array connected by lines and numbers indicating a particular sequence among them. The participant describes each picture in the route in order.

Choral reading
The clinician and the participant together read printed sentences.

Memory
An array of action pictures containing matching pairs is displayed for 30 seconds then the cards are turned over. On each turn, the participant turns over a card and describes it in a sentence, then looks for a match from memory, turns over another card and describes it. If a match is found, that pair is removed from the array.
Sentence completion
On each turn the participant completes a sentence stem presented orally by the clinician, to describe an action picture.

Generative protocol
There was no rehearsal or introduction of particular verbs prior to each activity. The participant was reminded of the sentence structure being used prior to the beginning of therapy and as necessary during treatment.

Picture description
The clinician and the participant are positioned on either side of a barrier to ensure the need for informative exchange and encourage verbal communication. Each has an identical set of pictures in front of her, but arranged in a random order. The participant selects one picture of the array and describes it using two different verbs in the target sentence structure. The clinician tries to select the picture that was described. The clinician and client take turns. After each picture description, the client and clinician reveal the picture they have each selected to see if they match.

"Go Fish"
The clinician and the participant are positioned on either side of a barrier to ensure only verbal communication is used. Participant and clinician play Go Fish as a language game using pictures. Three to seven pictures are dealt to each person from of a deck of picture pairs. The participant and the clinician take turns requesting a matching a picture using appropriate verbs in the target sentence structure.

Memory
An array of action pictures containing matching pairs is displayed for 30 seconds then the cards are turned over. The participant and clinician take turns describing from

memory and then selecting a likely location of matching picture cards using multiple verbs to describe each picture. If a match is found, that pair is removed from the array.

Story construction

The participant and the clinician take turns saying sentences to form a short story based on a single picture.

Map task

The clinician and the participant are positioned on either side of a barrier to ensure only verbal communication is used. The participant and the clinician each have in front of them a sheet of paper with multiple action pictures displayed in a random spatial pattern. The goal is for the participant to describe the route to the clinician (using two appropriate verbs to describe the action in each picture) so that the clinician can trace the identical route on her map. The participant and clinician take turns. After each map is described, the client and clinician reveal their maps to see if they have matching sequences.

Picture sequence

The clinician and the participant are positioned on either side of a barrier to ensure only verbal communication is used. The participant and the clinician have same stack of four or five unrelated picture cards in front of them in random order. The participant arranges her cards in a particular order and describes each picture (using two verbs) in the sequence she has arranged. The clinician attempts to mirror the sequence in her set of cards. The participant and clinician take turns. At the end of each series, the client and clinician reveal their picture sequences to see if they match.

APHASIOLOGY, 2011, 25 (11), 1347–1371

Monologues and dialogues in aphasia: Some initial comparisons

Elizabeth Armstrong[1], Natalie Ciccone[1], Erin Godecke[1], and Betty Kok[2]

[1]School of Psychology and Social Science, Edith Cowan University, Perth, Australia
[2]Department of Linguistics, Macquarie University, Sydney, Australia

Background: In recent years, there has been a shift in aphasia research interest from analysis of monologues to conversational dialogues. However, where monologic research has focused primarily on aspects such as language structure and quantity, conversational research has mainly focused on pragmatic aspects of discourse such as turn taking and repair. While there is some acknowledgement of the differences between language use in monologues and dialogues in aphasia, few comparisons have been made that cover a broad range of both syntactic and semantic aspects.
Aims: This study aims to compare the discourse of aphasic speakers and non-brain-damaged control speakers in monologues and dialogues by using a range of syntactic and semantic analyses. In so doing, it aims to explore whether or not it is necessary for researchers and clinicians to sample both contexts in order to gain a full picture of a person's linguistic skills.
Methods & Procedures: Two individuals with aphasia of varying severity provided monologues about their stroke experience, then participated in dialogues with a "significant other" on the same topic. Two control speakers, matched as closely as possible with the speakers with aphasia, undertook the same tasks, however they discussed a serious illness they had experienced. The SALT program (Miller & Iglesias, 2008) analysed the resulting data for syntactic productivity and complexity, and semantic analyses from a Systemic Functional Linguistic framework (Halliday & Matthiessen, 2004) were used to explore ideational, interpersonal, and textual meanings.
Outcomes & Results: The syntactic measures demonstrated greater consistency across contexts, with the participants with aphasia using more and longer C-units in the monologue, although demonstrating more mazes in this context. The control speakers demonstrated slightly more variation but, like the speakers with aphasia, tended to use more words per C-unit in the monologue. Semantic measures demonstrated more variable patterns although some similarities also existed.
Conclusions: The variation noted in the study supports the notion that clinicians and researchers should sample a variety of contexts in order to gain an overall picture of a person's language skills. Factors such as personality, topic, and conversation partner influence all seem to play a role in discourse production, particularly from the perspective of meanings conveyed. This study raises questions as to the actual effects of these

Address correspondence to: Prof. Elizabeth Armstrong, School of Psychology and Social Science, Edith Cowan University, 270 Joondalup Drive, Joondalup, Perth, Western Australia 6027, Australia. E-mail: b.armstrong@ecu.edu.au

http://dx.doi.org/10.1080/02687038.2011.577204

factors on language structure and function and provides direction for future research in the area.

Keywords: Aphasia; Monologue; Dialogue.

In recent years there has been a shift in the focus of aphasia research from analysis of purely monologic discourse to conversational dialogue as a source of data reflecting a person's language abilities in everyday interactions. This shift in attention developed from the need to understand the constituent parts of aphasic conversations in order to assist in remediation of conversational participation of people with aphasia. However, clinical assessment of discourse typically remains focused on monologic language samples largely gained from picture descriptions and story retells. This paper focuses on similarities and differences in the language produced in monologic and dialogic samples in order to explore the different sources of data and their respective contributions to clinical assessment.

Analysis of monologic discourse such as narratives has revealed much about aphasic difficulties in terms of macrostructural and microstructural organisation, and potential relationships between discourse skills and overall cognitive function. Aphasia is known to negatively affect lexical diversity, syntactic complexity, and cohesion during discourse production, while overall text macrostructure, pragmatic skills, and some aspects of evaluative language are relatively retained, if simplified, at least for people with mild and moderate aphasia (e.g., Armstrong & Ulatowska, 2007; Glosser & Deser, 1990; Gordon, 2006; Lock & Armstrong, 1997; Olness, Matteson, & Stewart, 2010; Ulatowska, North, & Macaluso-Haynes, 1981; Ulatowska & Olness, 2003). However, the linguistic skills of the person with aphasia during dialogue remain far less well understood. Studies emanating from a Conversation Analysis (CA) framework (e.g., Damico, Simmons-Mackie & Oeschlager, 1999; Heeschen & Schegloff, 2003; Simmons-Mackie & Damico, 2008; Wilkinson, Beeke, & Maxim, 2003) have added much to our understanding of the conversational dynamics in people with aphasia, and indeed have recommended that monologic narratives and casual conversational data are complementary and should be included in all clinical assessments (Beeke, Wilkinson, & Maxim, 2007). However, conversational studies to date tend to investigate more "pragmatic" aspects of conversation rather than the more syntactic and semantic aspects that have been the focus of monologic analyses. For example, monologic studies are typically concerned with "amount" of information conveyed, grammaticality and complexity of that information in syntactic terms, and discourse structure in terms of informational units such as orientation, complicating action, and resolution of narratives. CA studies, on the other hand, are typically concerned with the ways in which speakers negotiate meanings through repair and turn taking (Booth & Perkins, 1999; Simmons-Mackie & Damico, 2008), laughter (Oeschlager & Thorne, 1999), "speaking for" another (Croteau & LeDorze, 2006; Purves, 2009) and a variety of behavioural characteristics that are not necessarily related to linguistic structure per se.

Only a few studies have explored the aphasic speaker's grammatical functioning during conversation, and even fewer have looked at semantic aspects. Some studies that focused on agrammatism and telegraph-style speech (Heeschen & Schegloff, 1999; Kolk & Heeschen, 1990) have suggested that different patterns of grammar are demonstrated by individuals with Broca's aphasia between contexts such as picture descriptions and informal conversation. Indeed, Heeschen and Schegloff (1999, p. 374) suggest that: " . . . the use of telegraphic style is not only dependent on the situation in gross terms (such as testing vs. conversation), but also on the conversational partner, his/her interactional practices, and the tenor of the interaction at that moment."

Heeschen and Schegloff (1999) reported one speaker who attempted complete sentences while undertaking a picture sequence description, but who used "telegraphic" speech (utterances without finite verbs in particular) during an informal conversation. Beeke et al. (2003, 2007) have also demonstrated differences between uses of particular grammatical forms during testing/monologic discourse and conversation. They again report aphasic speakers using more complete grammatical forms during monologic discourse than conversation. Hence there is a small body of evidence suggesting that differences exist between language used in monologic tasks and that used during conversation in aphasic speakers. However, while these CA results focus on specific patterns of grammar, there are few studies that provide an overall picture of how linguistic patterns might vary across both syntactic and semantic measures that are compatible with both monologue and dialogue.

Jorgensen and Togher (2009) recently explored this issue in the area of traumatic brain injury. They had participants with TBI and non-brain-damaged control participants produce a narrative from a series of pictures, then produce a co-constructed narrative with a friend after both watching a video and having to convey the information to the naive researcher. Jorgensen and Togher reported the participants with TBI performed more like their non-brain-damaged counterparts during the co-constructed narrative than during the monologue on most measures, including C-unit productivity, cohesion, exchange structure, and story grammar. When comparing contexts, however, there were few differences between contexts except for the participants with TBI producing more story elements and more essential elements during the jointly produced narrative, although trends were also reported for a higher level of cohesion during the dialogue. The authors concluded that, for people with TBI, benefits of conversational support can be demonstrated.

In research investigating non-pathological discourse, while researchers acknowledge the difference between genres and contexts (e.g., Butt, Fahey, Feez, Spinks, & Yallop, 2000; Halliday & Matthiessen, 2004), there are again few studies that systematically explore the difference between one context and another in a way that is clinically accessible. One of the few studies directly comparing syntactic skills in two contexts explored the language of typically developing children and non-brain-damaged adults during expository discourse vs clinical conversations (Nippold, Hesketh, Duthie, & Mansfield, 2005). These authors reported on 40 adults (20 in the age range 20;8–28;5, and 20 in the range of 40;8–49;9). They measured syntactic complexity in terms of T-units, and their constituency in terms of independent and subordinate clauses. Nippold et al. reported no differences in overall number of T-units produced, a higher mean length of T-unit in expository discourse than during conversation, and a higher clausal density (i.e., no. independent clauses + subordinate clauses per T-unit) in the expository genre. It must be noted, however, that the conversations took place between the research participant and the researcher rather than a family member or friend, and from the description contained in the report it appeared that the conversation took the form more of an interview rather than a true informal conversation.

While the above studies have suggested that primarily syntactic differences exist between linguistic performance during monologue and dialogue, further data are required in order to address a broader measure of syntactic skills, *as well as* semantic issues. The lack of semantic analysis of discourse phenomena to date leaves a large gap in knowledge regarding the kinds of meanings people attempt to/are able to convey in different contexts and the kinds of wording used to convey such meanings. To date, investigations of semantics in discourse have predominantly either continued to focus on word-level contributions or have looked at overall discourse structure and coherence. For example, studies have examined the aphasic speaker's ability to use lexical items during spontaneous speech that have been taught as single words in treatment (e.g., Herbert, Hickin, Howard, Osborne, & Best, 2008; Hickin, Best, Herbert, Howard, & Osborne, 2001). Studies have also examined the aphasic speaker's ability to use elements of narrative structure such as orientation, complicating action, and resolution (e.g., Ulatowska et al., 1981), and establish coherence (Glosser & Deser, 1990; Olness, 2006). However, fewer studies have examined the speaker's ability to discuss different topics, provide opinions as opposed to simply factual information, or use different types of lexical items for different purposes, e.g., material and relational verbs to describe events, mental verbs to express positive or negative thoughts or feelings, emotive adjectives to express their perspective on events. Studies that have addressed these concerns (e.g., Armstrong, 2005; Armstrong & Ulatowska, 2007; Ferguson, Worrall, Davidson, Howe, & Sherratt, 2010; Olness et al., 2010; Ulatowska & Olness, 2003) have found that, while individuals with aphasia have retained some ability to convey emotional information and opinions, they are relatively restricted in this area when compared to their non-aphasic counterparts, especially in terms of variety and level of abstractness. However, these studies have not addressed such aspects of discourse in a conversational context, exploring the effects of conversational partners on the aphasic speaker's ability to create these meanings. Information gained from exploration of such aspects may well further inform hypotheses about processing of language during different contexts. In addition, clinicians need to be convinced that differences exist if they are to employ different methods from the currently typical default method of eliciting monologic discourse as the primary way of gauging a person with aphasia's linguistic skill level.

The current study is a preliminary exploration of both syntactic and semantic aspects of the discourse of people with aphasia during monologic narratives and conversation. Going beyond word-level semantics, this paper focuses on discourse semantics and meanings beyond individual word referents. It investigates whether differences occur in terms of frequency of different types of structures and meanings across the two contexts. It also provides a very preliminary exploration of the effects of different conversation partners, looking at potential interactional influences on the person with aphasia's expression. Two people with aphasia of differing severities and conversation partners, and two control speakers and conversation partners provide the data for the study. Exploration of two case studies with large speech sample size provides a good basis for initial quantification of potential similarities and differences.

METHOD

Participants

Two female participants with aphasia (PWA) were the focus of this study. They were both more than 5 years post stroke and had nonfluent aphasias. However, their severities differed. PWA1 was rated as a 4 on the Boston Diagnostic Aphasia Examination's Aphasia Severity Rating Scale (Goodglass & Kaplan, 1983) and PWA2 was rated a 2. PWA1 could carry on a conversation about most topics but was hesitant, took longer than normal to express ideas, and would sometimes get very frustrated looking for a word. PWA2 could also discuss a range of topics but had more difficulty, and often gave up on certain topics if she could not express herself. Additionally, the listener tended to share a lot of the burden in everyday conversations. The PWA were matched as closely as possible with two control speakers in terms of age, gender, and education/work background; and four non-brain-damaged conversation partners. For the dialogues, PWA1 and Control 1 (C1) spoke with their husbands of more than 20 years. PWA2, a widow, spoke with a female friend of a similar age while Control 2 (C2), also a widow, spoke with her granddaughter who was 40 years of age. Participant details are provided in Table 1.

Each PWA was initially asked by the researcher to provide a 10-minute recount of their experience of their stroke (their conversation partners were not in the room). Ten minutes is recommended as a representative sample of conversation (Boles, 1997) but constitutes a considerably long monologue, hence provides a monologic sample that is longer than most monologic discourse samples reported to date. The initial eliciting instruction was "Please tell me about your experience of your stroke – anything you'd like to tell me. I'd like you to talk for about 10 minutes if possible." If the speaker(s) indicated they were finished their discourse before the 10 minutes were completed, the researcher used prompt questions to facilitate further talking. These included

TABLE 1
Summary information about the participants with aphasia and their matched controls

	PWA[1]		*Control*	
	1	*2*	*1*	*2*
Age	65 years old	86 years old	62 years old	86 years old
Illness	Stroke	Stroke	MRSA	Macular degeneration
Gender	Female	Female	Female	Female
Time post illness	6yrs	9yrs	1.5 yrs	1yr
BDAE Aphasia Severity	4	2	N/A	N/A
Aphasia Type	Nonfluent	Nonfluent	N/A	N/A
Conversation partner	Husband	Friend (aged 86)	Husband	Grand daughter (aged 40)
Education level (PWA/C)	12 yrs	11 yrs	14 yrs	11 yrs
Employment (PWA/C)	Prior to stroke worked as national sales manager of international company	3 yrs clerical work after leaving school, then domestic duties	Nurse	Clerical work prior to retirement
Education level (Conversation partner)	10 yrs	11 yrs	10 yrs	14 yrs
Employment (Conversation partner)	"Estimator" for a fitting company prior to retirement	Domestic duties	Worked in bank for 38 years	High school teacher

[1]PWA = Person with aphasia.

"Can you tell me anything else?" or followed up on particular aspects of the recount. However, interaction with the participant(s) was kept to a minimum. A second sample was then obtained (with a 20-minute interval between samples) from the PWA and her conversation partner on the same topic. The conversation was elicited by the following instruction "I want you both to discuss X's stroke for around 10 minutes – anything you remember about it or to discuss about how it happened." The researcher remained in the same room but at a distance from the couple. The same procedure was used to elicit discourse from the control speakers except that they were asked to speak about a serious illness they had experienced. Control 1 (C1) discussed her experience of hospitalisation due to septicaemia, which was a complication of an MRSA infection. Control 2 (C2) discussed her treatment for macular degeneration. These speech samples were all collected at the participants' homes. Audio and video recordings were taken of the speech samples so that they could be transcribed for analysis.

The framework for analysis

Measures of overall productivity, grammatical complexity, and semantic content were included in the analysis. The productivity and complexity measures were included to reflect the lexical and structural aspects measured to date in monologic discourse studies, while the semantic measures were based on a Systemic Functional Linguistic (SFL) framework (Halliday & Matthiessen, 2004). This framework specifically addresses discourse-level semantics by exploring meanings that relate to overall textual meaning. The measures employed have been used in monologic discourse studies to date and have been demonstrated to be sensitive to the aphasic deficit. These are described, in detail, below.

Overall analytic procedure

Following orthographic transcription, the discourse samples were segmented into communication units (C-units). A C-unit is a main clause together with any subordinate clauses (Miller & Iglesias, 2008). While mazes ("repetitions, revisions, false starts and filled pauses"; Miller & Iglesias, 2008, p. 17) were included for the analysis of maze content, the words contained within mazes were excluded for all other analyses.

Productivity and complexity

The SALT (Miller & Iglesias, 2008) computer program was used to analyse the samples and calculate measures of productivity, specifically measures of linguistic complexity and completeness, as well as semantic diversity. For each discourse sample the measures used were:

- Number of C-units: the number of C-units included in the analyses.
- Percentage of C-units produced by focus speaker: Calculated within the dialogic speaking conditions this measure is the number of C-units produced by the study participant divided by the total number of C-units.
- Mean length of C-unit (words): the average number of words per C-unit.
- Type token ratio (TTR): the number of different words divided by the total number of words produced.

- Percentage of words in mazes (%words in mazes): the number of words contained within mazes divided by the total number of words.
- Number of abandoned C-units: the number of C-units that were voluntarily stopped, by the speaker, in the middle of the C-unit (Miller & Iglesias, 2008).
- Omissions/errors including omitted words, incorrect words and C-unit-level errors (Miller & Iglesias, 2008). Definitions provided by the SALT 2008 Instructional Version (Miller & Iglesias, 2008) were used for these measures. Omissions were marked if a word, required for the grammatical completeness of a C-unit, was omitted. A word-level error was marked if a word was used incorrectly and a C-unit-level error was marked when an error could not linked with a single word.
- The mean number of clauses per C-unit, including main and subordinate clauses.

The full discourse sample for each speaker was used for all of the above measures except for the calculation of TTR. As sample length has been shown to influence TTR (Wright, Silverman, & Newhoff, 2003) the samples were truncated to 200 words. The 200-word length was selected following the procedure of Wright et al. (2003) and excluded words contained within mazes.

Within the dialogic discourse samples, each of the above measures was calculated separately for each speaker.

Semantic content

While lexical diversity and word-level errors were tapped by the SALT analysis, further text-level semantic analyses were performed—specifically Transitivity, Appraisal, and Cohesion analyses. These constitute the three main types of meaning postulated in SFL: ideational, interpersonal, and textual meanings respectively, explained below. In addition a Topic Analysis (Mentis & Prutting, 1991) was performed in order to further highlight organisation of information structure.

The total data set was used for the Transitivity, Appraisal, and Topic analyses, but due to lack of reliability measures of cohesion analysis being available on lengthy texts such as the ones used in this study, the first 50 utterances of the focused speaker constituted the data for the Cohesion analysis. In the dialogues the individuals with aphasia PWA1 and PWA2, and the control speakers C1 and C2, were the focus of the analyses, although their contributions are depicted within the context of both conversational partners. In the cohesion analysis ties can obviously occur both between a speaker's own utterances and between her and her conversational partner's utterances. Both types of cohesive ties were analysed. The following provides detail of each analysis.

Transitivity. Transitivity (Halliday & Matthiessen, 2004) involves *ideational/informational meanings* related to the participants and actions constituting events being discussed. In particular, the verb is the focus of this analysis. The verb is purported to be the central meaning in the clause, conveying the nature of the activity being reported on, with specific verb patterns reflecting specific discourse genres (Butt et al., 2000). As analysis of semantic verb patterns has been found to be relevant to aphasic discourse (Armstrong, 2005; Berndt, Burton, Haendiges & Mitchum, 2002; Bird & Franklin, 1996; Edmonds, Nadeau, & Kiran, 2009), the Transitivity analysis was used to highlight the speakers' abilities to convey different types of ideational meanings in this study. The five major verb categories—material, mental, relational, verbal, and behavioural—were analysed to reflect the processes contained in clauses related to action, thinking/feeling, being, talking, and physiological processes such as breathing, coughing etc. These reflect the variety and patterns of meaning conveyed by the speaker (examples of different verb types produced by the speakers are given in Appendix A). Predominance of one verb type, e.g., material verbs, might reflect a relatively concrete recount where actions were the focus, as opposed to a recount where the speaker used a lot of mental verbs to reflect on events and portray feelings, or verbal verbs used to report specific things that were said.

Appraisal. Appraisal (Martin & White, 2005) focuses on *interpersonal meanings* conveyed through the use of evaluative language—language conveying emotions and opinions. These include both positive and negative connotations realised through words such as *lovely*, *terrible*, *hate*, *like*, and metaphoric utterances such as *I felt as if my life had blown away*. Such meanings go beyond the informational content typically counted in aphasic discourse, i.e., their ability to convey facts, and are crucial to a person conveying his/her identity. In this analysis the percentage of C-units containing evaluation was calculated, as well as the valence, i.e., the positive or negative nature of the evaluation. Evaluative language is felt to be a vital part of self-expression and is complementary to the ideational meanings outlined above. Measuring the valence of the evaluations (i.e., positive vs negative evaluation) is a further measure of addressing the type of meanings conveyed in each context. Examples of evaluative utterances and their valences produced by participants are given in Appendix B.

Cohesion. Cohesion (Halliday & Hasan, 1985, 1994) involves *textual meanings*, i.e., meanings involved in pulling the text together into a coherent whole. The texts were analysed for grammatical tokens and ties, e.g., pronouns /demonstratives and their referents, as well as the lexical relationships of antonymy, synonymy and other collocational relationships where words related to the same topic are expected to co-occur, creating continuity of topic (e.g., *well*, *sick*, *tired*, *energetic*, *stroke*, *illness* etc.). Following Halliday and Hasan's (1985) analysis, semantic "tokens" were initially identified throughout the texts. Tokens refer to content words or words taking the place of content words such as pronouns or demonstratives. Those tokens entering into a semantic relationship with another token (e.g., pronoun/referent relationship, synonymy, antonymy) were then put into cohesive chains, which represent the continuity of the text.

In the monologues the following phenomena were calculated, which reflect the amount of continuity in the text:

1. Total number of tokens.
2. Total number of cohesive chains.
3. Total number of tokens in cohesive chains.
4. Total tokens in cohesive chains as a percentage of total tokens in the text.
5. Number of cohesive "errors": grammatical cohesive markers such as pronouns and demonstratives were counted as incomplete or erroneous if no clear referent could be found in the surrounding text, as described by Liles and Coelho, 1998; lexical markers such as "one" and "thing" denoting non-specific referents were also noted as incomplete or erroneous if no clear referent could be established.

During a dialogue, cohesion can occur across one speaker's utterances as well as between speakers. Hence the following measures aimed to capture the speaker of interest's contribution to any chains formed within the dialogue, and to capture the person's ability to enter into interactive chains with the other speaker. In the dialogues, the following phenomena were calculated:

1. Total number of tokens (i.e., including both speakers).
2. Total number of cohesive chains (both speakers).
3. Number of interactive chains (i.e., cohesive chains containing contributions from both speakers).
4. Number of total tokens in cohesive chains (both speakers).
5. Speaker of interest's (i.e., individuals with aphasia or controls) total number of tokens.
6. Speaker of interest's (i.e., individuals with aphasia or controls) number of tokens in cohesive chains.
7. Speaker of interest's (i.e., individuals with aphasia or controls) number of tokens in cohesive chains as a percentage of their total tokens.
8. Number of cohesive errors.

An example of cohesive chaining is given in Appendix C.

Topic structure

In order to determine the depth of information provided by speakers, a topic analysis (Mentis & Prutting, 1991) was used, which gave a broad overview of the different aspects of events recounted in the monologic and conversational samples. As the main topic of the discourse samples was stipulated (as per task instructions above), the number and nature of the introduced subtopics was the focus of this analysis. Subtopics were outlined by Mentis and Prutting (1991) as embedded subtopics and defined as follows: "those subtopics in which the focus of discussion . . . was part of and germane to the main topic sequence" (p. 585). The subtopic was a subordination of the main topic and was either an elaboration or expansion of the main topic. The total number of subtopics, the number of introductions per speaker, and mean number of C-units per subtopic (per speaker) were calculated from the discourse samples. An example of topic analysis is given in Appendix D.

Reliability

The transcripts were checked by a second analyst and any differences resolved prior to analysis. The productivity/complexity analyses were undertaken using the automated SALT analyses, hence they were consistent and replicable.

Inter-rater reliability for each of the semantic measures undertaken was calculated, based on 25% of the data being analysed by a second analyst. The results were as follows. In terms of categorisation of verbs used by participants in the transitivity analysis, inter-rater agreement was 85%. In terms of number of C-units identified as containing evaluation, 86% agreement was reached. Rating of valence achieved 100% agreement. For the cohesion measures, the following levels of agreement were obtained:

1. Total number of tokens: 82%.
2. Total number of chains: 84.5%.
3. Total number of tokens in cohesive chains: 82.5%.
4. Number of cohesive "errors": 100%.

RESULTS: PWA1 AND C1

Productivity and complexity

In terms of the amount and complexity of language produced across contexts, PWA1 produced more C-units in the monologue than in the dialogue, an unsurprising result since the samples were each 10 minutes in length and a dialogue would lessen opportunities for production in terms of amount of speech produced by one speaker. As indicated by percentage of C-units produced within the dialogue, PWA1 and C1 produced a similar number of C-units to their communicative partners (see Table 2). The mean length of PWA1's C-units in words was higher in the monologue, and her C-units contained marginally more clauses within the monologue. The percentage of words in mazes was higher in the monologue, as were number of errors produced. However, PWA1's TTR was similar across contexts.

C1 produced more C-units within the monologue, contributing an equal number of C-units as her communicative partner within the dialogic sample. Her mean length of C-unit was slightly higher in the monologue sample while the mean number of clauses per C-unit was slightly higher in the dialogue. C1's TTR was similar across contexts. However, similar to PWA1, the amount of words within mazes was higher in the monologue.

In terms of overall comparison between PWA1 and C1 in each context, they differed on six out of the eight measures analysed. While the number of C-units produced by each was similar in the monologue, C1 produced more C units in the dialogue than PWA1. C1's mean length of clauses and mean number of clauses per C-unit were higher in both contexts, PWA1 had a higher overall percentage of words in mazes than C1, and while PWA1's texts contained word omissions and errors, C1 did not demonstrate these at all. C1's TTRs were also higher than PWA1's in both contexts.

Transitivity. PWA1 demonstrated use of all verb types overall, but demonstrated a different pattern between the contexts. There was a predominance of material and relational verbs in the monologue, with fewer mental and verbal verbs and no behavioural verbs. PWA1 hence produced both a factual recount and descriptive recount involving evaluations through relational verbs such as "*it was good*", but did not use many actual mental verbs in conveying direct feelings e.g., "*I felt* . . . .". In the dialogue material verbs still predominated, but relationals were used less than in the monologue and mentals were used more. This corresponds to the more direct reference to feelings by

TABLE 2
PWA1 and C1: Productivity and complexity results

	PWA1 Monologue	*PWA1 Dialogue*	*C1 Monologue*	*C1 Dialogue*
#C-units	101	44	105	68
Mean Length of C-Unit (wds)	6.92	4.84	10.25	9.51
Mean # Clauses per C-unit	1.06	1.02	1.64	1.69
% C-units contributed	100%	52%	100%	51%
TTR	0.46	0.47	0.54	0.52
% wds in mazes	22%	14%	8%	4%
#Abandoned C-units	3	3	3	3
#Omitted words/errors	17	4	0	0

TABLE 3
PWA1 and C1: Transitivity results

	PWA1 Monologue	PWA1 Dialogue	C1 Monologue	C1 Dialogue
Material	54 (45%)	18 (52%)	66 (40%)	37 (34%)
Relational	53 (44%)	11 (31%)	69 (41%)	39 (36%)
Mental	5 (4%)	6 (17%)	25 (15%)	23 (21%)
Verbal	8 (7%)	0	4 (2%)	7 (6%)
Behavioural	0	0	3 (2%)	3 (3%)
Total	120	35	167	109

PWA's partner, who asked his wife on several occasions how she felt after the stroke, hence increasing the potential number of mental verbs used. C1 showed more consistency across contexts, with material and relational verbs predominating in both the monologue and dialogue, although to a slightly lesser degree in the dialogue. The dialogue was very interactive, and both discourse samples were relatively factual and descriptive rather than involving much discussion of feelings. These results are summarised in Table 3

Comparing PWA1 and C1 overall, C1 tended to use fewer material verbs and more mental verbs than PWA1. C1 also demonstrated use of all verb types, while PWA1 did not produce any behavioural verbs, and verbal verbs only in the monologue context.

Evaluation

PWA1 was consistent across contexts, producing a similar number of C-units containing evaluation. C1's use of evaluation was also similar across contexts (see Table 4).

In terms of valence PWA1 demonstrated similar patterns across contexts, with both being more positive than negative. However, quantitatively PWA1 tended to be more positive during the monologue than the dialogue (69% in the monologue; 53% in dialogue). This may be related to PWA1's husband's contributions, which were mainly negative in valence, i.e., pointing out the negative life changes as a result of PWA1's stroke. In response PWA1 acknowledged and elaborated on these more during the dialogue than the monologue, where she presented a more positive stance. C1 also had a consistent pattern across contexts, but evaluations were more negative than positive in both contexts (60% negative in monologue and 60% in dialogue). This pattern most likely occurred because PWA1 was discussing a stroke and was taking the perspective of how she has managed to get on with her life in a positive way. Conversely, C1's

TABLE 4
PWA1 and C1: Evaluation results as percentage of C-units containing evaluation and percentage positive and negative valence

	PWA1 Monologue	PWA1 Dialogue	C1 Monologue	C1 Dialogue
C-units containing evaluation	35 (36%)	15 (34%)	30%	25%
Positive valence	69%	53%	40%	40%
Negative valence	31%	47%	60%	60%

experience was that of a transitory illness, where the experience itself was a negative one and was the focus of the conversation, rather than the "recovery." Overall, PWA1 used more evaluation than C1.

Cohesion

PWA1 had similar levels of cohesion in both texts and in fact contributed to 60% of the dialogue's overall cohesion. She demonstrated only a small number of problematic tokens, with slightly more occurring in the dialogue. During the dialogue PWA1's husband led a lot of the conversation, prompting her at different points—e.g., prompting her to remember places they had been for holidays—but PWA1 was certainly able to participate in joint chains with her husband, sometimes initiating these herself, with interactive chains (chains involving both conversation partners) constituting 72% of all cohesive chains. C1 had slightly less cohesion in the dialogue. However, C1 contributed less to the overall cohesion of the dialogue than did PWA1. PWA1's husband tended to facilitate PWA1's contribution through his prompting and questions, and hence could have facilitated her cohesion in this way. As C1's conversation partner largely controlled the conversation in terms of the illness narrative, it may be that he dominated the cohesion as well. Of the chains in the overall text, 50% were interactive, indicating that several cohesive chains were created by the partners independently. This reflects the different speakers' independence in contributing different aspects of their experience. These results are summarised in Tables 5 and 6. Overall comparisons reveal instances of problematic use of cohesive devices are higher in the PWA's discourse, and that patterns of chain construction and interaction differ between the PWA and the Control speaker.

Topic structure

The monologues contained more subtopics for both PWA1 and C1 than the dialogues but both used more C-units per topic in the dialogue (see Table 7). PWA1 in fact introduced all the subtopics in the monologue, whereas C1 had to be prompted by the researcher for several subtopics. Both depended on the other speaker more in the dialogue. It could be hypothesised that the familiarity of the conversation partner facilitated more in-depth discussion of each subtopic and encouraged both PWA1 and C1 to produce more utterances. However, this is speculation only, as quantitative measures such as "subtopic" and "C-units per subtopic" may be interpreted in different ways. For example, more subtopics and fewer C-units per subtopic may mean that a

TABLE 5
Cohesion results for PWA1 and C1 monologue

	PWA1	*C1*
#Tokens	162	248
#Tokens in chains	121	200
%Tokens in chains	75%	81%
#Chains	20	29
#Incomplete/errors	4	1

TABLE 6
Cohesion results for PWA1 and C1 dialogue

	PWA1	*C1*
#Total tokens	297	477
#Tokens in chains	219	350
#PWA/C total tokens	131	225
#PWA/C tokens in chains (% of total PWA/C tokens)	100 (76%)	160 (71%)
%PWA/C tokens in chains of total tokens in chains in text	60%	46%
#Chains overall	36	60
#Interactive chains	26 (72%)	30 (50%)
#Incomplete/errors	5	1

TABLE 7
Topic results for PWA1 and C1

	PWA1 Monologue	*PWA1 Dialogue*	*C1 Monologue*	*C1 Dialogue*
Total subtopics	15	6	12	8
No. subtopics introduced	15	2	5	2
Mean #C-units per subtopic	7	8.3	9	9.5

person is elaborating on a broader range of subtopics (different aspects of the experience), but is not elaborating in very much depth. Fewer subtopics and more C-units may mean that the person is elaborating on particular aspects in more depth. Both constitute a form of elaboration of the overall topic and it is difficult to place a value on this, although people with aphasia may be compensating by using a greater number of subtopics in order not to have to explore depth of one aspect of the discourse. In terms of overall differences between PWA1 and C1, the main difference was that overall, C1 produced more C-units per subtopic than PWA1, while in the monologue, PWA1 generated more topics and subtopics independently.

RESULTS: PWA2 AND C2

Productivity and complexity

PWA2 produced a similar pattern to PWA1 except that the number of C-units was similar across the two contexts. Her mean length of C-units in words was higher in the monologue, and her C-units contained more clauses within the monologue than the dialogue. Her TTR was similar across contexts. Percentage of words in mazes was higher in the monologue, as were number of omitted words and word errors (see Table 8).

C2 used a similar number of C-units across contexts, but used fewer words in the dialogue. Her mean length of C-unit in words was similar across contexts, but the mean number of clauses was higher within the dialogue. TTR was similar across contexts. Mazes occurred more often in the monologue and there were few lexical errors in either context. Comparisons between PWA2 and C2 overall again revealed differences on six of the eight measures. Number of C-units was higher for C2 in the monologue, mean length of C-units overall was higher for C2, as was mean number of clauses per

TABLE 8
PWA2 and C2: Productivity and complexity results

	PWA2 Monologue	*PWA2 Dialogue*	*C2 Monologue*	*C2 Dialogue*
#C-units	90	93	103	92
%C-units contributed to dialogue		48%		48%
Mean length of C-unit(wds)	7.70	5.57	8.54	8.10
Mean #Clauses per C-unit	1.37	1.08	1.42	1.46
TTR	0.44	0.47	0.50	0.47
%Wds in mazes	20%	15%	5%	2%
#Abandoned C-units	14 (13%)	18 (14%)	6	7
#Omitted words/errors	16	9	1	0

C-unit. While TTRs were similar, percentages of words in mazes, abandoned C-units and frequency of word omissions and other errors were all higher for PWA2.

Transitivity. PWA2 demonstrated a variety of verb types across contexts. She used predominantly material verbs in both, reflecting her more concrete recount overall, however she used significant amounts of relational, mental, and verbal verbs in the monologue. A similar pattern was demonstrated in the dialogue. C2 demonstrated a more different pattern of usage across contexts by increasing her usage of material verbs in the dialogue context and decreasing her use of relational and mental verbs. This reflected the more factual nature of the dialogue as elaborated on below (see summary of results in Table 9). Overall, C2 tended to use more relational and mental verbs than PWA2.

Evaluation. PWA2 used less evaluation during the dialogue (6%) than the monologue (19%), as did C2 (see Table 10). PWA2 was relatively factual in both recounts, but her personality was a very practical one (as reported by family and

TABLE 9
PWA2 and C2: Transitivity results

	PWA2 Monologue	*PWA2 Dialogue*	*C2 Monologue*	*C2 Dialogue*
Material	47 (38%)	41 (44%)	34 (23%)	59 (40%)
Relational	26 (21%)	25 (26%)	55 (37%)	36 (24%)
Mental	24 (20%	16 (17%)	44 (30%)	33 (22%)
Verbal	25 (20%)	12 (13%)	4 (3%)	12 (8%)
Behavioural	1 (1%)	0	11 (7%)	8 (6%)
Total	123	93	148	148

TABLE 10
PWA2 and C2: Evaluation results as percentage of C-units containing evaluation and percentage positive and negative valence

	PWA2 Monologue	*PWA2 Dialogue*	*C2 Monologue*	*C2 Dialogue*
C-units containing evaluation	17 (19%)	6 (6%)	38 (37%)	24 (26%)
Positive valence	59%	16%	50%	46%
Negative valence	41 %	74 %	50 %	54 %

friends) and premorbidly she might not have been a person who spoke about her feelings very much. However, the fact that she used less evaluation in the dialogue than in the monologue perhaps occurred because of less opportunity for evaluation, and more reliance on the conversational partner. The partner really mainly contributed sympathetic comments on what PWA said rather than inducing or encouraging her to express further evaluation, for example:

10. Partner: [And where were you when it happened
11. PWA2: And I was at home
12. Partner: Oh that was [terrible
27. PWA2: I just said I can't speak anymore
28. Partner: Oh yes that was [shocking

C2 used more evaluation than PWA2 but, as noted above, tended to give more of her own feelings in the monologue, and focus more on factual elements during the dialogue with her granddaughter as they recounted events surrounding the eye treatment being discussed.

PWA2 demonstrated much more positive evaluation during the monologue than the dialogue. In the monologue she tended to focus more on how good her recovery had been and that she was "lucky" in many ways and also tended to minimise the extent of her difficulties:

64. I was not I was coping all right til the other day
65. but then I got another little stroke.
66. R: Right [Researcher]
67. But it wasn't very much
79. You know very mild stroke
96. and I learned because I I learned learned to speak on the phone straight and straight away because I couldn't I had to so many friends that uh I learned to speakers on the phone
97. and a lot of people can't speak on the phone
98. but I just kept on speaking uh my my cousins and things like that
99. I did them better.
100. Then X gave me quite a lot of lessons which I was very pleased
110. I was very lucky that the family was with me

Similar to PWA1, the relative negativity of the dialogue could have been influenced by her conversation partner who predominantly gave sympathetic comments regarding the difficulties associated with the stroke and the event itself—e.g. *that's shocking, that must have been terrible* etc. In fact PWA2 used the word *terrible* on a couple of occasions, and was also accredited for co-construction of evaluation through ellipsis, e.g., the conversation partner said: *Isn't that strange* and PWA2 replied *Yes.*

In terms of valence, C2 used equal amounts of positive and negative evaluation in the monologue and slightly more negative evaluation in the dialogue (54% negative).

Cohesion. PWA2 had similar levels of cohesion in both contexts and contributed 60% of the overall cohesion of the dialogue—largely composed, however, of repetition of lexical items and information. She was able to co-construct cohesion with her partner, as 59% of the overall chains in the text were interactive. PWA2 demonstrated 12 instances of problematic cohesion in the monologue, while she only had 3 instances in the dialogue. While PWA2 said fewer overall words in the dialogue this was not proportional to her errors, hence it did appear that monologue produced relatively more

TABLE 11
Cohesion results for PWA2 and C2 monologue

	PWA2	*C2*
#Tokens	216	226
#Tokens in chains	166	148
% Tokens in chains	77%	65%
#Chains	23	26
#Incomplete/errors	12	0

TABLE 12
Cohesion results for PWA2 and C2 dialogue

	PWA2	*C2*
#Total tokens	246	370
#Tokens in chains	188	292
#PWA/C total tokens	138	219
# PWA/C tokens in chains (% of total PWA/C tokens)	113 (82%)	162 (74%)
% PWA/C tokens in chains of total tokens chains in text	60%	55%
# Chains overall	27	38
#Interactive chains	16 (59%)	27 (71%)
#Incomplete/errors	3	3

errors. C2 demonstrated slightly less cohesion in the dialogue and contributed slightly less to the overall cohesion of the dialogue. However, interactive chains made up 71% of the total chains in the dialogue. She demonstrated no incomplete ties in the monologue but had three problematic instances in the dialogue. Results are summarised in Tables 11 and 12.

Overall comparisons reveal higher numbers of cohesive tokens in PWA2's chains. However, the contribution of repetition to PWA2's cohesion is acknowledged above. A higher number of interactive chains by Cl is noted above in terms of the dialogue.

Topic structure

PWA2 and C2 showed the opposite pattern from their counterparts in that they demonstrated more subtopics in the dialogues (see Table 13). They also showed more utterances per subtopic in the monologue rather than the dialogue. Again the issue of familiarity of partners and, in particular, shared experience might have limited the depth of subtopic discussion in the dialogue, leading to a greater range of subtopics and fewer utterances related to them. PWA2 demonstrates a slightly smaller mean

TABLE 13
Topic results for PWA2 and C2

	PWA2 Monologue	*PWA2 Dialogue*	*C2 Monologue*	*C2 Dialogue*
Total subtopics	8	13	7	13
No. subtopics introduced	2	5	4	5
Mean #C-units per subtopic	11.8	9.8	15	8.2

number of utterances per subtopic in the monologue than C2, indicating less elaboration and extension of the main topic when compared within the dialogue. PWA2 had slightly more C-units per subtopic than the matched control when speaking in a shared communicative interaction (dialogue). This indicates that, in their respective dialogue samples, PWA2 contributed at least the same level of topic maintenance as C2 within a familiar topic.

The similarity between PWA2 and C2 is interesting given the severity of PWA2's aphasia. However, it has to be noted that it has been more than 5 years since PWA2's stroke—she has been successful in reintegrating into social situations and has regained her ability to participate in conversations. Hence, even though her linguistic structure is affected, she retains the ability to introduce and maintain topics. No overall differences between the speakers in terms of topic were noted, except for the relatively higher number of C-units per subtopic in the monologue by C2.

DISCUSSION

In exploring the contexts of monologue and dialogue, this study highlights aspects of discourse that can both potentially change and remain similar across contexts. The results raise issues related to the effects of aphasia severity, familiarity between conversation partners, personal style, and topic. While these factors have been raised previously as being potentially influential in discourse construction, the current study explores the type of specific language issues that may be affected by such factors. The study also raises issues related to quantification of meaning and individual variability, and the need to incorporate such issues into standard clinical assessments.

Overall the detailed analysis showed wide variation between speakers across contexts, although some areas demonstrated similarity as well. It appears also that syntactic features may be more consistently affected by context than semantic features, which can be affected differentially by the multiple factors just mentioned.

Productivity

In terms of productivity and complexity it appears that both people with aphasia were able to produce more language and with greater complexity during monologues. This is consistent with previous findings (e.g., Beeke, Wilkinson, & Maxim, 2003; Heeschen & Schegloff, 2003). However, they also had more words in mazes and more errors in the monologues, which would suggest that dialogue provides some scaffolding for processing. The control speakers demonstrated more consistency across contexts, although they also demonstrated more mazes in the monologues, reinforcing the notion that even non-brain-damaged speakers' processing may be assisted or at least masked/facilitated in a dialogue situation where there is assistance from a partner and also perhaps more context provided because of this. A priming effect is also a possible explanation of these results. As the speech samples were obtained with only a minimal interval between them, it is possible that processing was assisted in the dialogue through speakers' prior processing of concepts, lexical items, and structures related to an identical topic during the monologue context. While this is a potential explanation in light of the overall topic being the same, the differences in the content and tone of the monologues and dialogues reflect the fact that this was not a case of someone undertaking an identical task on two closely situated occasions.

Meanings conveyed were often quite different, with conversation partners in the dialogue often eliciting quite different aspects of the situations under discussion. Another aspect worth raising here is the equal contribution in C-units of each speaker to the dialogue. Future studies might include a measure of the amount of time occupied by each speaker within the 10-minute dialogue as not only an indication of content contribution, but also a reflection of processing time required for this content. Such a measure may well reveal a difference in the "contribution" of aphasic versus non-aphasic speakers.

Transitivity

The variation that occurred across contexts for two of the four speakers was not easily explained. C1 and PWA2 were the most consistent. In PWA2's case one could speculate that she tended to use a similar pattern of verb meanings across both monologue and dialogue due to lexical restrictions for particular verb categories, hence there was less chance of variation as she was the more impaired aphasic speaker. However, as noted, C1 also had a similar pattern across contexts. Partner influence expressed itself in different ways. For example, PWA1's husband asked specific questions potentially leading PWA1's verb usage, whereas for some reason C2 and her granddaughter co-constructed a more factual account of her eye disease than C2 had given alone. This could have been due to a number of factors, e.g., that neither person wanted to elaborate so much on the emotional aspect when the other was present, that the granddaughter was not involved as closely in the event and hence tended to focus on the facts, etc. In terms of consistency across contexts the partners (or their presence) may also have had an influence, e.g., PWA2's partner was fairly passive in the dialogue, largely making sympathetic comments, hence PWA2 used much the same resources to tell the story as when she was doing this alone. However, C1's partner was quite active in the conversation and, as they had experienced the illness together, had a similar way of describing it to the way in which C1 expressed the events alone.

Evaluation

Evaluation patterns were similar across monologue and dialogue for PWA1 and C1 but differed for PWA2 and C2, although the latter two varied in the same direction, i.e., more in the monologue than the dialogue. This difference between pairs could be related to different level of familiarity of the speakers' conversational partners. The two husbands were the most familiar and had shared the experience with the PWA and the Control speaker, hence they were potentially more emotionally involved in the recount of events. This meant that both contexts tended to be relatively emotionally charged. This differed from PWA2 and C2 whose partners hadn't been through the experience with them and who, while both acknowledging feelings, tended to share less of their own feelings or inquire of the person's feelings at the time. For example, while PWA2's partner was very sympathetic, she tended to ask factual questions of her.

Of note here is the relative lack of evaluation by PWA2 in the dialogic context. Her level of evaluation is lower than her control speaker and lower than PWA1, potentially reflecting her greater aphasia severity and potential difficulty with the abstractness required for reflection/evaluation, as well as premorbid personality. However, while she is able to produce evaluative comments in the monologue, she produces none in the dialogue. As mentioned, this could reflect either a dependence on her conversation partner who provided much evaluation, or difficulty in producing more abstract comments during a faster-flowing dialogue. The valence, however, was of interest. The people with aphasia tended to be more positive in their monologues than in the dialogues, with their conversational partners tending to focus on the negative aspects of the stroke, rather than the people with aphasia conveying their optimism to the independent person (the researcher). The control speakers, on the other hand, tended to be more consistent across contexts, with negative evaluation reflecting their negative experience of an illness, but not one that required long-term recovery and adjustment in the same way as a stroke involves.

Cohesion

While the aphasic speakers demonstrated similar amounts of cohesion across contexts, the control speakers demonstrated differences. C1 was more cohesive in the monologue while C2 was more cohesive in the dialogue. There is no obvious reason for this, other than to speculate on individual processing differences. For example, C1 might have been more focused on topic during the monologue than the dialogue, which was more dominated by her partner, whereas C2 might have depended more on the partner's contributions to create her cohesion. One of the issues in quantifying cohesion is that aspects such as repetition are potentially counted as cohesive, hence aphasic speakers who tend to have restricted lexical variety might have falsely inflated cohesion counts because of this. This was true of both PWA1 and PWA2, so more in-depth analysis would have to be provided in order to tease out the contributions of phenomena such as repetition. However, it is interesting that the supposed scaffolding of the other speaker during the dialogue would not have increased their cohesion further. Again, further analysis of the quality and subpatterns of cohesive device usage may shed further light on the nature of the cohesion exhibited by the individuals with aphasia. Cohesive "errors" were noted in all speakers' texts, although minimally in the control and PWA1's texts. PWA2, however, did demonstrate a reasonable number of errors in the monologue, suggesting that, when left to her own resources, cohesion did suffer more than when she had a conversation partner for scaffolding. Alternatively, a priming /rehearsal effect may also be a potential explanation for this finding.

Topic structure

The topic structure analysis provides a good example of the difficulties in attempting to quantify semantics. As noted in the Results section, quantity of units, such as subtopics, does not really indicate the quality of these units. A higher number of subtopics does not necessarily guarantee better elaboration of a topic. It could be that, for people with aphasia, fewer subtopics and more utterances would assure better clarity. On the other hand, more subtopics introduced, i.e., different aspects of an event, may in fact be a good strategy if the speaker is unable to elaborate on these aspects through multiple turns. At least the speaker is attempting to provide a variety of meaning within the discourse.

Nevertheless the results indicate that both people with aphasia were able to produce a significant number of topics independently, and that both produced differing amounts between the two contexts. This suggests that, in the clinical assessment setting, a speaker could either be under- or over-estimated (in terms of what s/he is able to talk about) if only sampled in one context.

General conclusions

Meanings will potentially be more variable than syntactic structures, and perhaps it may be impossible to look for consistent patterns of meaning across speakers of the types explored in this paper. However, in order to explore natural language use, clinicians and researchers alike need to explore variability as much as trying to minimise variation for the purposes of measurement. While measurement issues are crucial for aspects of clinical work such as monitoring effects of treatment/improvement etc., analyses that highlight a person's total linguistic and communicative resources are also crucial if we are to gain a realistic picture of someone's communicative functioning.

It is difficult to extricate patterns from two case studies. Further studies in this area obviously need more participants in order to explore potential patterns that may become more evident across a group of speakers. However, in-depth description of each of the semantic analyses reported above, which was beyond the scope of this paper, may also reveal patterns that may be useful in beginning to understand contextual, interpersonal, and intrapersonal variation.

The study has raised more questions than it answers, but in so doing provides a challenge for further exploration of semantic aspects of discourse. While word and sentence phenomena tell one part of the linguistic story, information on semantics at the discourse level is needed in order to bridge the gap between current word-based accounts of discourse and the more recent CA approaches to largely pragmatic aspects of conversation management. The analyses used in this study align with suggestions made by both Jorgensen and Togher (2009) in the area of TBI and Sherratt (2007), who advocate for multi-layered examinations of discourse in order to uncover the intricacies of everyday communication. Discourse involves the interaction of numerous syntactic, semantic, and pragmatic elements of language, and while all these aspects are inherent in monologue, dialogue complicates the picture even further. Frankel and Penn (2007) have pointed out that conversation is a complex endeavour requiring considerable executive function skills such as planning, sequencing, monitoring, attention, as well as linguistic skills, and that numerous such factors operating in conversation will potentially affect a speaker's ability to access and utilise available language resources. Hence there is much work to be done to uncover how language works during conversation and to examine the significance of conversational dynamics in influencing linguistic usage. These initial comparisons of monologue and dialogue may begin to shed light on this issue. The findings are important in highlighting the subtle scaffolding and influence that takes place in conversations between people with aphasia and their family members or conversation partners. This is important considering the increasing trend in therapy to include family members or focus treatments on the dyad.

The differences found in the data reported here suggest that speakers may vary across contexts and that this variation should be expected to some extent in everyday discourse. Variability in performance has been suggested as being a feature of aphasia (Cameron, Wambaugh, & Mauszycki, 2010; Kolk, 2007). However, its presence in the discourse of non-brain-damaged speakers and the potential effects of communication partners are often overlooked when variability is approached as if it is pathological in nature, rather than a normal phenomenon. While potential priming/rehearsal effects must also be considered in the interpretation of some of the results presented here, many of the patterns could not be explained from this perspective, and attest to the multiple factors potentially affecting dialogic discourse production in particular.

The further exploration of such factors in clinical assessments of individuals with aphasia is hence essential if the clinician is to get a true picture of the speaker's overall linguistic skills.

REFERENCES

Armstrong, E. (2005). Expressing opinions and feelings in aphasia: Linguistic options. *Aphasiology*, *19*(3/5), 285–296.

Armstrong, E., & Ulatowska, H. K. (2007). Making stories: Evaluative language and the aphasia experience. *Aphasiology*, *21*(6/7/8), 763–774.

Beeke, S., Wilkinson, R., & Maxim, J. (2003). Exploring aphasic grammar 2: Do language testing and conversation tell a similar story? *Clinical Linguistics and Phonetics*, *17*(2), 109–134.

Beeke, S., Wilkinson, R., & Maxim, J. (2007). Grammar without sentence structure: A conversation analytic investigation of agrammatism. *Aphasiology*, *21*(3/4), 256–282.

Berndt, R. S., Burton, M. W., Haendiges, A. N., & Mitchum, C. C. (2002). Production of nouns and verbs in aphasia: Effects of elicitation context. *Aphasiology*, *16*(1/2), 83–106.

Bird, H., & Franklin, S. (1996). Cinderella revisited: A comparison of fluent and non-fluent aphasic speech. *Journal of Neurolinguistics*, *9*(3), 187–206.

Boles, L. (1997). Conversation analysis as a dependent measure in communication therapy with four individuals with aphasia. *Asia Pacific Journal of Speech, Language and Hearing*, *2*, 43–61.

Booth, S., & Perkins, L. (1999). The use of conversation analysis to guide individualized advice to carers and evaluate change in aphasia: A case study. *Aphasiology*, *13*(4/5), 283–303.

Butt, D., Fahey, R., Feez, S., Spinks, S., & Yallop, C. (2000). *Using functional grammar: An explorer's guide*. Sydney: Macquarie University.

Cameron, R., Wambaugh, J., & Mauszycki, S. (2010). Individual variability on discourse measures over repeated sampling times in persons with aphasia. *Aphasiology*, *24*(6–8), 671–684.

Croteau, C., & LeDorze, G. (2006). Over-protection, "speaking for", and conversational participation: A study of couples with aphasia. *Aphasiology*, *20*(2/3/4), 327–336.

Damico, J. S., Simmons-Mackie, N., & Oeschlager, M. (1999). Qualitative methods in aphasia research: Conversation analysis. *Aphasiology* *13*(9/10/11), 667–680.

Edmonds, L. A., Nadeau, S. E., & Kiran, S. (2009). Effect of Verb Network Strengthening Treatment (VNeST) on lexical retrieval of content words in sentences in persons with aphasia. *Aphasiology*, *23*(3), 402–424.

Ferguson, A. J. (1998), Conversational turn-taking and repair in fluent aphasia. *Aphasiology*, *12*(11), 1007–1031.

Ferguson, A., Worall, L., Davidson, B., Howe, T., & Sherratt, S. (2010). Talk about our goals for aphasia therapy: A systemic functional analysis. *Journal of Interactional Research in Communication Disorders*, *1*(1), 95–118.

Frankel, T., & Penn, C. (2007). Executive dysfunction as an explanation for conversation symptoms of aphasia: A pilot study. *Aphasiology*, *21*(6/7/8), 814–828.

Glosser, G., & Deser, T. (1990). Patterns of discourse production among neurological patients with fluent language disorders. *Brain & Language*, *40*, 67–88.

Goodglass, H., & Kaplan, E. (1983). *Boston Diagnostic Aphasia Examination*. Philadelphia: Lea & Febiger.

Gordon, J. K. (2006). A quantitative production analysis of picture description. *Aphasiology*, *20*(2–4), 188–204.

Halliday, M. A. K., & Hasan, R. (1985). *Language, context and text: Aspects of language in a social-semiotic perspective*. Geelong, Australia: Deakin University Press.

Halliday, M. A. K., & Hasan, R. (1994). *Cohesion in English*. London: Longman.

Halliday, M. A. K., & Matthiessen, C. M. I. M. (2004). *An introduction to functional grammar* (3rd ed.). London: Arnold.

Heeschen, C., & Schegloff, E. (1999). Agrammatism, adaptation theory, conversation analysis: On the role of so-called telegraphic style in talk-in-interaction. *Aphasiology*, *13*, 365–405.

Heeschen, C., & Schegloff, E. (2003). Aphasic agrammatism as interactional artifact and achievement. In C. Goodwin (Ed.), *Conversation and brain damage* (pp. 231–282). New York: Oxford University Press.

Herbert, R., Hickin, J., Howard, D., Osborne, F., & Best, W. (2008). Do picture-naming tests provide a valid assessment of lexical retrieval in conversation in aphasia? *Aphasiology*, *22*(2), 184–203.

Hickin, J., Best, W., Herbert, R., Howard,D., & Osborne, F. (2001). Treatment of word retrieval in aphasia: Generalisation to conversational speech. *International Journal of Language & Communication Disorders*, *36*(Supplement), 13–18.

Jorgensen, M., & Togher, L. (2009). Narrative after traumatic brain injury: A comparison of monologic and jointly-produced discourse. *Aphasiology, 23* (9), 727–740.
Kolk, H. (2007). Variability is the hallmark of aphasic behaviour: Grammatical behaviour is no exception. *Brain and Language, 101*, 99–102.
Kolk, H. H. J., & Heeschen, C. (1990). Adaptation symptoms and impairment symptoms in Broca's aphasia. *Aphasiology, 4*, 221–231.
Liles, B., & Coelho, C. (1998). Cohesion analyses. In L. Cherney, B. Shadden, & C. Coelho (Eds.), *Analyzing discourse in communicatively impaired adults*. Gainsburg, MD: Aspen Pub.
Lock, S., & Armstrong, L. (1997). Cohesion analysis of the expository discourse of normal\fluent aphasic and demented adults: A role in differential diagnosis? *Clinical Linguistics & Phonetics, 11*(4), 299–317.
Martin, J. R., & White, P. R. R. (2005/2007). *The language of evaluation: Appraisal in English*. Basingstoke, UK: Palgrave Macmillan.
Mentis, M., & Prutting, C. A. (1991). Analysis of topic as illustrated in a head-injured and normal adult. *Journal of Speech and Hearing Research, 34*, 583–595.
Miller, J., & Iglesias, A. (2008). *Systematic Analysis of Language Transcripts (SALT), Instructional Version 2008* [computer software]. Madison, WI: University of Wisconsin-Madison, Waisman Research Center, Language Analysis Laboratory.
Nippold, M. A., Hesketh, L. J., Duthie, J. K., & Mansfield, T. C., (2005). Conversational versus expository discourse: A study of syntactic development in children, adolescents, and adults. *Journal of Speech, Language, and Hearing Research, 48*, 1048–1064.
Oeschlager, M., & Thorne, J. C. (1999). Application of the Correct Information Unit Analysis to the naturally occurring conversation of a person with aphasia. *Journal of Speech, Language, & Hearing Research, 42*, 636–648.
Olness, G. S. (2006). Genre, verb, and coherence in picture-elicited discourse of adults with aphasia. *Aphasiology, 20*(2–4), 175–87.
Olness, G. S., Matteson, S. E., & Stewart, C. T. (2010). "Let me tell you the point": How speakers with aphasia assign prominence to information in narratives. *Aphasiology, 24*(6–8), 697–708.
Purves, B. (2009). The complexities of speaking for another. *Aphasiology, 23*(7/8), 914–925.
Sherratt, S. (2007). Multi-level discourse analysis: A feasible approach. *Aphasiology, 21*(3/4), 375–393.
Simmons-Mackie, N., & Damico, J. S. (2008). Exposed and embedded corrections in aphasia therapy: Issues of voice and identity. *International Journal of Language and Communication Disorders, 43*(S1), 5–17.
Ulatowska, H., & Olness, G. (2003). On the nature of direct speech in narratives of African Americans with aphasia. *Brain and Language, 87*, 69–70.
Ulatowska, H. K., North, A. J., & Macaluso-Haynes, S. (1981). Production of narrative and procedural discourse in aphasia. *Brain and Language, 13*, 345–371.
Wilkinson, R., Beeke, S., & Maxim, J. (2003). Adapting to conversation: On the use of linguistic resources by speakers with fluent aphasia in the construction of turns at talk. In C. Goodwin (Ed.), *Conversation and brain damage* (pp. 59–89). New York: Oxford University Press.
Wright, H. H., Silverman, S. W., & Newhoff, M. (2003). Measures of lexical diversity in aphasia. *Aphasiology, 15*(5), 443–452.

APPENDIX A

Examples of different verb types

Material verbs (actions):
I was admitted to hospital
He couldn't take me to theatre
They lanced it
He came
My neighbour took me to the hospital

Mental verbs (affect/cognition):
They decided that it was an abscess
Other people must feel terrible
The surgeon saw me
I thought I'm just lucky
I wanted some things

Relational verbs (verbs of "being/existing"):
It was quite a large cavity
It was MRSA
I had a large lump there
I'm lucky
It's good

Verbal verbs (talking):
The surgeon said
I couldn't speak at all
He asked her
The doctor suggested I get them done
I often say

Behavioural verbs (physiological):
My nose runs
I tighten up
I couldn't sleep
Just relax

APPENDIX B

Examples of evaluative utterances

I would like to have them here	*POSITIVE*
You're very nice	*POSITIVE*
And I frustrating	*NEGATIVE*
In temperament you're a bit different	*NEGATIVE (IN CONTEXT OF TEXT)*
It really went downhill from there	*NEGATIVE*
I felt like a leper I guess	*NEGATIVE*
It was a bit of a joke	*NEGATIVE*
And that was even worse	*NEGATIVE*

APPENDIX C(I)

Sample analysis of excerpt from PWA1 dialogue (C-units 9–20): Transcript and rendering of tokens for cohesion analysis

9	D	What's the major change do you feel
10	PWA1	uh well well because my grandchildren everything
11	PWA1	I I I would like to have them here
12	PWA1	But I can't have them here anymore
13	D	Because you can't really look after them way you used to
14	PWA1	Not um Dylan now he's six
15	PWA1	And he he he's older
16	PWA1	But um Nathan and Benjamin and Mitchell get on with their lives anyway
17	PWA1	where where what did you what is the first thing the that I did you did think of just
18	D	Well I think the major change is you can't do things you used to ten years ago
19	D	So you can't travel freely the same way as you could
20	D	If you want board aircraft that's difficult

Rendering of tokens from the text

C-Unit			*Number of tokens*
9	D	major change you feel	4
10	PWA1	my grandchildren	2
11	PWA1	I have them here	4
12	PWA1	I have them here	5
13	D	you look-after them you look-after	6
14	PWA1	Dylan he is six	4
15	PWA1	He is older	3

16	PWA1	Nathan Benjamin Mitchell get-on their lives	6
17	PWA1	thing I think	3
18.	D	I think major change is you do things you do ten-years-ago	11
19	D	You travel	2
20	D	you travel you travel	4
21	D	You want board aircraft that be difficult	7

APPENDIX C(II)

Cohesive chains

9 D major
18 D major

8 D change
18 D change

11 L have
12 D have

10L Grandchildren
11L them
12L them
13D them
14L Dylan
15L he
16L he
17L Nathan
18L Benjamin
19L Mitchell

11L here
12L here

14L is
15D is
128. D is

5 D look-after
D look-after

14 L six
15 L older

9 D you
10 L my
11 L I
12 L I
13 D you
13 D you
17 L I
18 D you
18 D you
19 D you
20 D you
20D you
21 D you

17L think
18L think

19 D travel
20 D travel
20 D travel

APPENDIX D

Sample analysis of excerpt from PWA1's monologue: Topic analysis

SubTop	*SubTop*	*C-unit*
		Now the the 15th of april 1999 I had a stroke
1		And I we went to the mall
		Uh that's warringah mall here
		And I just fell down just fell down
		And then I had an ambulance
	2	and get um
		the doctor said to me well I'd what what is it
		And I said oh I can't speak very well
		And then hehey went to my up my up to my husband
		and everybody came
		Everybody came
3		And then um um I went to the upstairs the hospital
		and then I had a BIG stroke {L facial grimace}
		A very very bad
		but it doesn't matter now
		It's done and dusted {L laughs}
	4	Um and uh I went to uh nine days after I went to Coorabel
		and it was good good in there
		Um and I had about uh uh seven eight nine weeks ne nine weeks
5		and and it's not it's not very good
		But it doesn't matter now because nine uh nine years later just get on with it
		Get on with it {L laughs, gesture with hand of moving forward}
	6	And um um I was a little bit teary and everything because um the I I I came home and I could/'t speak
		I could speak um yes and no
		that's all I could speak
		but um later got a little bit better
7		Um uh um Don he he he's uh he's very he's fantastic with me
		but he doesn't {L laughs} he doesn't he does guts frustrated for a while
		And and then and then he hehe's very nice to me
		and and he he doesn't he doesn't
		he's he's seventy two seventy three now

APHASIOLOGY, 2011, 25 (11), 1372–1392

A multi-level approach to the analysis of narrative language in aphasia

Andrea Marini [1,2], Sara Andreetta[1], Silvana del Tin[3], and Sergio Carlomagno[4]

[1]Dipartimento di Scienze Umane, University of Udine, Udine, Italy
[2]IRCCS "E. Medea: La Nostra Famiglia", San Vito al Tagliamento (Pn), Italy
[3]IMFR Gervasutta, Udine, Italy
[4]Dipartimento di Psicologia, Università di Trieste, Trieste, Italy

Background: Several studies have shown that traditional standardised aphasia tests may not be sensitive enough to adequately assess linguistic deficits and recovery patterns in persons with aphasia. As a result, both functional and structural methods for the analysis of connected language samples from people with aphasia have been devised (see Armstrong, 2000; Prins & Bastiaanse, 2004).
Aims: The present article focuses on our attempt to provide a comprehensive, multi-level procedure for both structural and functional analysis of narrative discourse produced by speakers with brain damage. Accordingly, we will describe a method for analysis of connected language samples elicited on single picture and cartoon story description tasks. This method has proven sensitive in the assessment of language deficits in many neurogenic populations.
Methods & Procedures: A comprehensive description of the language production system, a thorough discussion of the different approaches to discourse analysis in persons with aphasia, and the procedure for the analysis of narrative discourse are detailed. The characteristics of the eliciting stimuli, the procedures for their administration and the transcription of the language samples are carefully explained. The analysis focuses on four main aspects of linguistic processing: productivity, lexical and grammatical processing, narrative organisation, and informativeness. To further illustrate the analytic procedure, two case reports and an appendix with the analysis of a narrative sample are provided.
Outcomes & Results: We will provide direct evidence of the usefulness of the multi-level procedure for discourse analysis for assessing changes in discourse performance of two persons with fluent aphasia, with different aetiologies, that were not captured by traditional standardised aphasia tests.
Conclusions: The method of analysis presented in this paper has strong grounds in linguistic and psychological theories of linguistic structure and functioning. It also has the advantage of being both quantitative and functional as it captures selective

Address correspondence to: Andrea Marini PhD, Università di Udine, Via Margreth, 3 – 33100 Udine, Italy. E-mail: andrea.marini@uniud.it

The authors are indebted to Dr Alessia Granà for the careful assessment of the participants with standard aphasia tests before and after the therapy. They wish to thank Angy Perkins-Schmitt for the linguistic revision of the paper. Finally, the authors are grateful to the two anonymous reviewers for their insightful comments to the first version of the paper.

http://dx.doi.org/10.1080/02687038.2011.584690

aspects of linguistic processing, and can provide relevant information about the person's communicative and informative skills.

Keywords: Neuropsychology; Aphasia; Language; Narrative analysis.

In the last three decades a growing interest in the way language is processed in daily communicative interactions (i.e., spontaneous language) has challenged the traditional views of how to assess language deficits in persons with aphasia (PWA). An important premise of this change in perspective is the increasing awareness that traditional standardised aphasia tests may not be sensitive enough to adequately assess linguistic deficits and recovery in these persons. For example, it has been noted that examination of spontaneous language according to traditional aphasia assessment batteries provides clinicians with very limited information about the interaction among several processing levels such as those between verb processing, argument structure generation, sentence production, and inter-utterance integration (e.g., Armstrong, 2000; Prins & Bastiaanse, 2004; Saffran, Berndt, & Schwartz, 1989; Shewan, 1988). Larfeuil and Le Dorze (1997) analysed the patterns of language recovery of a cohort of 17 PWA. At 17 weeks post-onset and after 6 weeks of language stimulation therapy, these persons were given standardised aphasia tests and a picture-description task for eliciting a sample of narrative discourse. In this study the standardised aphasia assessment failed to show any improvement.

However, the analysis of the language samples that were gathered during the pre- and post-therapy assessment showed an improvement in communicative effectiveness as measured in terms of production of open-class words per time unit. In a similar vein, Helm-Estabrooks and Ramsberger (1986) analysed the recovery patterns of a group of persons with chronic agrammatic aphasia receiving intensive therapeutic interventions aimed at improving their morpho-syntactic and syntactic skills. Pre- and post-therapy assessments were evaluated using a picture description task (Cookie Theft picture; Goodglass & Kaplan, 1972). The multi-level analysis of discourse performance showed that, after therapy, the participants had better morphosyntactic skills resulting in more informative speech (for a similar procedure see also, Rochon, Saffran, Berndt, & Schwartz, 2000). In a previous study by our group (Marini, Caltagirone, Pasqualetti, & Carlomagno, 2007) three individuals with non-fluent aphasia, whose speech was characterised by reduced information content and poor morpho-syntactic organisation, received two consecutive therapy programmes. The first programme consisted of stimulus–response exercises for producing well-formed sentences (HELPSS; Helm-Estabrooks, Fitzpatrick, & Barresi, 1981). This was followed by a functional treatment programme in PACE format (Carlomagno, Losanno, Emanuelli, & Casadio, 1991) aimed at increasing their informativeness in storytelling. During the three assessments (before and after HELPSS and after modified PACE), the three participants were asked to describe two cartoon stories and two single pictures. These samples of connected speech underwent both linguistic and functional analysis in order to examine the patterns of their language recovery. Following the therapy programmes, only minimal changes were observed on standard aphasia tests (e.g., Aachener Aphasie Test, AAT, Italian version; Luzzatti, Willems, & DeBleser, 1991). However, the informativeness of the language samples increased and this improvement was recognised by non-expert judges. This suggests that the functional improvement was not due to increased syntactic abilities (see also Springer, Huber, Schlenck, & Schlenck, 2000). These findings clearly highlight the need for an assessment that jointly focuses on both structural linguistic and functional aspects of language processing. This would assist in evaluating residual discourse processing abilities, selecting candidates for specific therapy programmes, evaluating language improvement, and examining relationships between therapeutic programmes and patterns of recovery.

The present article focuses on our attempt to provide a comprehensive, multi-level procedure for the analysis of narrative discourse produced by brain-damaged speakers. Accordingly, we will outline a method for the analysis of language samples elicited during single picture and cartoon story description tasks. This method has proven sensitive in the assessment of language deficits not only in PWA (Marini, Caltagirone, et al., 2007) but also in other neurogenic populations including persons with right hemisphere damage (Marini, Carlomagno, Caltagirone, & Nocentini, 2005), traumatic brain injury (e.g., Carlomagno, Giannotti, Vorano, & Marini, 2008), schizophrenia (e.g., Marini, Spoletini, et al., 2008), children with specific language impairment (Marini, Tavano, & Fabbro, 2008) or with Williams' syndrome (Marini, Martelli, Gagliardi, Fabbro, & Borgatti, 2010), and people suffering from Duchenne muscular dystrophy (e.g., Marini, Lorusso, et al., 2007). These studies were also aimed at expanding on previously described methods for structural and functional analysis of narrative language (e.g., Haravon, Obler, & Sarno, 1994; Saffran et al., 1989; Shewan, 1988) and to assess patterns of language impairment in persons with and without aphasia. This allowed us to collect data from people without brain damage in order to detect changes in discourse processing during normal aging (Marini, Boewe, Caltagirone, & Carlomagno, 2005). It also allowed us to progressively revise the method in order to obtain measures that are reliably sensitive to damage to different components of the discourse processing system. For this reason an overview of the language production system will be provided to justify methods for both functionalist and structuralist discourse analysis in PWA (for comprehensive reviews on the argument see also Armstrong, 2000; Prins & Bastiaanse, 2004). Then two examples of the analysis applied to individuals with fluent aphasia will be discussed. Finally, an appendix will outline details of the analysis to familiarise the reader with the procedures of transcription and analysis.

AN OVERVIEW OF THE LANGUAGE PRODUCTION SYSTEM

Language is a complex dynamic cognitive system based on the integration of multiple competences along two main dimensions of processing (Caplan, 1992; Glosser & Deser, 1990): a within-utterance or micro-linguistic dimension, responsible for intra-sentential functions; a between-utterance or macro-linguistic dimension, responsible for inter-sentential functions. Importantly, the levels of language are deeply interconnected (e.g., Jakobson, 1980). The *micro-linguistic dimension* organises phonological or graphemical patterns into morphological strings and words (lexical processing) and determines the syntactic context each word requires for the generation of well-formed sentences (syntactic processing). The *macro-linguistic dimension* determines the contextually appropriate meaning of a word or a sentence (pragmatic processing) and connects sentences or utterances by means of cohesive and coherent devices in order to formulate the main theme of narrative discourse and integrate its linguistic and conceptual features (discourse processing; see Kintsch, 1994; Kintsch & van Dijk, 1978). Cohesion refers to the structural and semantic relations among contiguous utterances (cohesive ties: Halliday & Hasan, 1976). It is established through the use of both grammatical (e.g., pronouns, adverbs, definite articles, conjunctions, ellipsis, substitutions) and lexical (e.g., repetitions, synonyms, antonyms) cohesive markers. A cohesive marker is a word that ties the meaning expressed in the ongoing utterance with those already expressed, or those in planning, and to be expressed in the subsequent utterances. As such, cohesive markers establish meaning relationships across sentences within the passage. Cohesion violations occur when the referent of the information provided within a sentence is not readily available (van Leer & Turkstra, 1999). Disrupted cohesion may reflect a deficit in lexical retrieval (i.e., a micro-linguistic process) rather than impaired macro-linguistic organisation. Therefore it is plausible that cohesion connects micro-linguistic and macro-linguistic processes (Halliday & Hasan, 1976; see later for a detailed description of this link). Finally, global coherence refers to the ability to semantically relate remote utterances in the framework of a given discourse. Increasing evidence shows that micro- and macro-elaborative levels of language processing can be analysed separately (e.g., Davis, O'Neil-Pirozzi, & Coon, 1997).

This is the static picture of the language system. We will now examine the dynamics of the language production process. The currently accepted models appear to include at least three stages (Frederiksen, Bracewell, Breuleux, & Renaud 1990; Indefrey & Levelt, 2000, 2004; Levelt, 1989; Levelt, Roelofs, & Meyer, 1999): a pre-linguistic conceptual phase; a phase of linguistic formulation; and a phase of linguistic expression (e.g., articulation) where production actually takes place. In the pre-linguistic conceptual phase the speaker generates a mental model of the message he/she wants to produce. In doing this, he/she must retrieve the appropriate conceptual frame structure from long-term episodic memory (e.g., selecting the appropriate discourse genre). Then this structure must be filled with the semantic information (e.g., participants, setting, etc.) that pertains to the intended message. The speaker needs to integrate what he/she wants to say with what has been previously said (linguistic context), together with the particular situation, place and time in which the communicative exchange takes place (extra-linguistic context; Johnson-Laird, 1980; Levinson, 1983). This allows the speaker to regulate the amount of information that he/she intends to communicate and its relevance with respect to what has been previously said (Grice, 1975; Sperber & Wilson, 1986). This conceptual information triggers the generation of appropriate propositions that must be organised at the macro-linguistic level by means of adequate cohesion and coherent links.

In the *linguistic formulation phase* the preverbal message is converted into a speech plan. Here, lexical processing matches the intended meaning, formulated in the pre-linguistic phase, with the corresponding lexical items stored in the mental lexicon. This operation is performed through a multi-stage process that entails a phase of lexical selection and one of lexical access. The process of lexical selection allows the speakers to select the lexical items that correspond to the intended meanings (Levelt et al., 1999). How this selection takes place is still not completely clear. It is likely to be achieved through an activation/inhibition mechanism. Each word has its own specific activation thresholds as a function of the frequency of its use and time elapsed since last activation: The lower the threshold level, the easier the access; the higher the threshold level, the more difficult the access. The activation of the target word is achieved through the co-occurring inhibition of semantically related competitors. This inhibition may be obtained by raising the competitors' activation thresholds. If the speaker intends to say "apple", the activated concept corresponding to the idea of APPLE enters the lexicon. Here a selection mechanism is needed to properly select the target word ("apple") among all other semantically related lexical items ("pear", "orange", "banana", etc.). The activation threshold of the competitors is raised and the target word ("apple") is selected. At the end of the lexical selection process, the target word has been activated. The formulator gains access to its morphosyntactic and morphological features (lemma level of word representation) and then to its syllabic and phonological form. In the case of single word production, the lexical information is then transmitted to the output system where articulatory configurations corresponding to the phonemes to be uttered are programmed and then implemented. In the case of sentence production, such as in connected speech, the process of lexical selection and the access to a word's lemma form the "functional level" of sentence processing. Here, the morphosyntactic information required by the selected word (i.e., its argumental structure) guides the process of sentence generation by means of thematic roles' assignment and phrase generation. At the second level of sentence processing, the so-called "positional level", the information contained in the lemmas of the selected words is used to generate the grammatical relations among the phrases and to build up well-formed syntactic representations (Chomsky, 1995; Garrett, 1980). It is now possible to access the syllabic and phonologic representation(s) of the selected word(s). This information is eventually sent to the output system where articulatory configurations corresponding to the phonemes to be uttered are programmed and then implemented (*phase of linguistic expression*).

STRUCTURALIST APPROACHES TO DISCOURSE ANALYSIS IN PERSONS WITH APHASIA

From a structuralist/quantitative point of view, discourse is considered a complex structure made up of constituents at different levels of processing (i.e., phonological, lexical, grammatical, discourse; e.g., Saffran et al., 1989; Schwartz Saffran, Fink, Myers, & Martin, 1994). Several techniques have been described to elicit language samples from persons with brain damage. These include picture descriptions (e.g., Nicholas & Brookshire, 1993), story (re-)tellings (e.g., Saffran et al., 1989; Ulatowska, North, & Macaluso-Hayes, 1981), recounts of personal information (e.g., Glosser & Deser 1990), or descriptions of procedures (e.g., Ulatowska, Freedman-Stern, Doyel, Macaluso-Haynes, & North, 1983). The narrative discourse produced by an individual with aphasia may be analysed with quantitative measures of phonological processing, lexical selection, grammatical construction, and ability to provide adequate structural (cohesion) and semantic (coherence, both local and global) connections between the utterances.

Prins and colleagues (Prins, Snow, & Wagenaar, 1978; Wagenaar, Snow, & Prins, 1975) analysed the connected speech of unselected adults with aphasia on a variety of measures, such as speech rate, mean length of utterance, percentage of complex utterances, phonemic and verbal paraphasias, fluency, telegraphic speech, grammatical errors, articulation, and empty speech. A factor analysis revealed clustering of these variables on six factors: Fluency, Telegraphic speech, Grammatical errors, Articulation, Paraphasias, and Empty Speech (see also Vermeulen, Bastiaanse, & van Wageningen, 1989, for comparable results). These analyses, however, are time consuming and require a thorough knowledge of linguistics and aphasia. Therefore they are not routinely used in clinical practice. Another method was developed by Saffran and colleagues in 1989 to analyse the agrammatic speech of persons with Broca's aphasia. This method focused on measures of syntactic accuracy such as proportion of verb inflections, closed-class words, and well-formed sentences. Further methods of quantitative structural analysis of connected speech have been devised by Shewan (1988) and Obler and colleagues (Haravon et al., 1994). Mayer and Murray (2003) accurately demonstrated the usefulness of quantitative analysis of spontaneous speech obtained in PWA using a picture description task and a conversation about familiar topics. The authors demonstrated that three measures of word retrieval derived from discourse analysis (% Word Retrieval, % Substantive Verbs, and % Corrected Errors) differed significantly from the score obtained on a naming task. Both % Word Retrieval and % Corrected Errors were higher in connected speech than in naming. Furthermore, the % Substantive Verbs and the % Word Retrieval were found to be sensitive measures of possible verb retrieval deficits for people with mild aphasia (see also Prins & Bastiaanse, 2004, for a discussion of this issue). These results, together with data from the analysis of language samples from persons with agrammatism, indicate the relevance of quantitative measures of discourse. On the other hand, Ulatowska and colleagues (1981, 1983) analysed the narratives produced by PWA with respect to those produced by participants without brain damage. Overall, persons with both mild and moderate aphasia produced shorter and grammatically simpler narratives but elicited the essential elements of the story structure preserving the chronological order of events (Ulatowska et al., 1981, 1983). The studies of narrative production of PWA appeared to support the notion of a micro-linguistic impairment associated with relatively spared macro-linguistic abilities. Of course, this general assumption does not necessarily imply that all macro-linguistic skills are unimpaired in these individuals. Bloom, Borod, Santschi-Haywood, Pick, and Obler (1996) reported normal cohesive levels in the language samples from a group of PWA, and Glosser and Deser (1990) reported a group of individuals with fluent aphasia who showed lower levels of cohesion and coherence than healthy participants. Interestingly, they interpreted the reduced ability to provide adequate cohesive ties among utterances as a consequence of a deficit in lexical retrieval rather than a real problem in intersentential organisation (see also Bates, Hamby, & Zurif, 1983). It is often reported that PWA have difficulties in correctly linking adjacent utterances by means of adequate cohesive ties. For example, they have been found to use pronouns more often without antecedents (e.g., Glosser & Deser, 1990; Ulatowska et al. 1983, 1981). It remains controversial as to whether these errors are due to pragmatic deficits, or are an epiphenomenon of their lexical deficit (e.g., Bates et al., 1983; Christiansen, 1995; Glosser & Deser, 1990).

FUNCTIONALIST APPROACHES TO DISCOURSE ANALYSIS IN PERSONS WITH APHASIA

The functionalist approaches to discourse processing abilities in aphasia have mainly focused on the ability to convey information (e.g., Armstrong, 2000). One procedure for quantifying information content was originally developed by Yorkston and Beukelman (1980). They administered the Cookie Theft Picture description task (Goodglass & Kaplan, 1972) to a group of PWA. The levels of informativeness of these language samples were quantified in terms of Content Units (CUs), CUs per minute (CUs/m'), and Syllables per minute (Syllables/m'). A CU was defined as a grouping of information that had been mentioned by at least 1 of the 78 healthy individuals who had participated in the study. The number of CUs discriminated only between healthy participants and those with moderate aphasia, whereas the two measures of communicative efficiency (i.e., CUs/m', and Syllables/m') also discriminated between healthy participants and those with mild aphasia. The measures could even discriminate between different severity levels of aphasia. The CU analysis has proved useful for quantifying informativeness in PWA with high inter-rater reliability (> .90). Nonetheless, the method has undergone significant revisions. For example, Nicholas and Brookshire (1993) introduced the Correct Information Unit (CIU) analysis system. Correct Information Units (CIUs) represent words in the sample that are "accurate, relevant and informative relative to the eliciting stimuli" (Nicholas & Brookshire, 1993, p. 340). This method uses both quantitative and functional measures. Quantitative measures include the number of words and CIUs in the sample.

Functional measures include Words per minute, CIUs per minute, and the percentage of words in the sample that convey appropriate information (% CIUs), which is a new parameter of discourse efficiency not included in the CU analysis by Yorkston and Beukelman (1980). These measures have been shown to have high diagnostic sensitivity even in persons with mild fluent aphasia (Nicholas & Brookshire, 1993). Importantly, this system has good ecological validity, as changes in CIU measures of information content are perceived even by naïve listeners (Jakobs, 2001; Ross & Wertz, 1999). Furthermore, the CIU procedure has been applied to the analysis of several types of language samples elicited, not only with the Cookie Theft Picture but also with other stimuli—e.g., the WAB picture (Kertesz, 1982), picture sequences arranged in a story (Nicholas & Brookshire, 1993), procedural discourse and descriptions of personal events (Doyle, Goda, & Spencer, 1995; Nicholas & Brookshire, 1993). The CIU method, as used for the analysis of the efficiency of connected speech, seems to also have good test–retest reliability (> .88; Brookshire & Nicholas, 1994). This holds true in tasks where language samples are obtained with picture or cartoon-story descriptions, procedural discourse, and requests for personal information. However, Oelschlaeger and Thorne (2000) found lower inter-rater reliabilities for both CIUs and %CIUs (.54 and .39, respectively) when participants were asked to provide personal information.

More recently, Sherratt (2007) examined the interaction between the structural and functional aspects of narrative and procedural discourse. In this experiment each of the 32 non-brain-damaged participants was asked to produce up to 14 language samples, which included four narratives generated by picture sequences, four narratives related to personal experiences, and six procedures. These language samples were analysed in terms of seven broad features (comprising 23 measures), relating to the levels of the multi-level discourse model (i.e., relevance, discourse grammar, clarity disruptors, productivity and syntactic complexity, clausal structure, cohesion, and fluency). A series of correlations showed that many of these measures interact. For example, greater relevance was related to more appropriate discourse grammar, fewer non-specific elements, greater cohesion and syntactic complexity. Overall, the findings from this study suggest that a multi-layered approach to discourse analysis may prove useful in the assessment of linguistic skills of persons without and, possibly, with communication disorders, providing an additional perspective on how the different elements of a discourse interact.

A METHOD FOR THE ASSESSMENT OF MICRO- AND MACRO-LINGUISTIC SKILLS IN PERSONS WITH FLUENT APHASIA

Here, we will outline a method for the assessment of micro- and macro-linguistic skills in people with neurological or neuropsychiatric disorders which allows clinicians to derive both quantitative and functional measures. For example, we argue that this multi-level procedure for discourse analysis may provide important information about the linguistic skills of persons with fluent aphasia.

Stimuli

Four picture stimuli (two single picture scenes and two picture sequences, respectively) were used to obtain the discourse samples. These were selected to elicit samples ranging from 300 to 400 words, which is important for test–retest reliability (Nicholas & Brookshire, 1993). These stimuli also allow control over several factors that may affect discourse production. In addition, picture descriptions have elicited more grammatically analysable utterances and a similar range of elicited grammatical structures from people with aphasia as was produced in unstructured interviews (Easterbrook, Byers Brown, & Perera, 1982). The two single picture scenes we used were the "Cookie Theft" picture (Goodglass & Kaplan, 1972) and "The Picnic" (Western Aphasia Battery, WAB; Kertesz, 1982). The two picture sequences used are the "Flower Pot" (Huber & Gleber, 1982) and the "Quarrel" (Nicholas & Brookshire, 1993).

Administration of the stimuli and transcription of the samples

Each participant was asked to describe the situation in each of the four stimuli. The participants were told that there was no correct way to describe them, that they should avoid using ambiguous words, and that the administrator was not familiar with the story. The stimuli were administered using a laptop facing the participant to avoid short-term memory limitations and to avoid referent sharing. The samples were audio-recorded and transcribed verbatim including phonological fillers, pauses, false starts, and extraneous utterances. The duration of each sample was also calculated.

Linguistic analysis

This analysis focused on four main aspects of linguistic processing: productivity, lexical and grammatical processing, narrative organisation, and informativeness.

Productivity. Productivity measures included counting units and words, and computing speech rate and Mean Length of Utterance (MLU). The *unit* count included all verbalisations, irrespective of their linguistic or contextual correctness or appropriateness. Therefore particular care was taken to include in the unit count not only phonologically well-formed words, but also non-words (e.g., neologisms and phonological paraphasias), false starts, sounds, and syllable repetitions. The *word* count included only phonologically well-formed words, i.e., excluding phonological fillers and phonological errors. The number of words was used to obtain a measure of *speech rate* in terms of words per minute. For each story description the total number of *utterances* was calculated. Several criteria have been formulated to segment language samples into utterances (e.g., Shewan, 1988). For example, utterance boundaries have been determined by analysing intonation contours, grammatical completeness, and the presence of pause lengths. In our experience, however, it is hardly possible to provide a coherent segmentation by adopting just one criterion. We have identified a set of parameters that may variably account for utterance segmentation that has gained high inter-rater reliability scores. We have jointly adopted acoustic, semantic, grammatical, and phonological criteria. According to the *acoustic criterion* an utterance is an emission of sounds delimited by pauses that can be easily identified and may be either empty (such as silence) or full (non-lexical emissions such as "ehm" or fillers such as "I think", or "Let me guess"). Let's consider the following sequence: "this is a . . . [silent pause of 5 seconds] child". In this case, since a clear pause can be perceived between the first chunk "this is a" and the second one "child", the sequence can be segmented in two distinct utterances: / This is a . . . (5 seconds) / child /. According to the *semantic criterion* an utterance is a conceptually homogeneous piece of information—i.e., a proposition, defined as a semantic unit consisting of the main predicate with its arguments and all embedded predicates and argument(s) associated with it (Olness, Matteson & Stewart, 2010). Therefore, if there is not a sensible pause in the flow of speech, utterance boundaries can be identified whenever a proposition has been formulated and a new one is introduced. For example, the sequence "A man is walking on the road. A flower pot falls on his head" can be split in two distinct utterances: / A man is walking on the road / A flower pot falls on his head / because the second utterance introduces a new proposition. Similar considerations can be applied to the following utterances: / A man is walking on / He is running on the sidewalk / where the first proposition has not been completed and the second block provides a reformulation of the preceding one. According to the *grammatical criterion* for utterance segmentation, a block of words is an utterance when, in absence of clear pauses (acoustic criterion) and of propositional violations (semantic criterion), it forms a grammatically complete sentence (eventually also including subordinate clauses). In this case, even if long, the sequence can be considered a single utterance, as shown in the following example: / The man is walking on the sidewalk with a dog that looks very nice /. Nonetheless, if the speaker utters two coordinated sentences, these can be divided in two separate utterances: / The man is walking on the sidewalk / and a dog is following him /. This is because the utterance count is important for several derived measures capturing grammatical, cohesive and coherent aspects of linguistic processing. According to the *phonological criterion* if a word is interrupted (i.e., there is a false start), then the utterance is considered abruptly interrupted as well. For example, in the following sequence: / and she is ca- / stroking his d- / his d- / the dog of the the man / four distinct utterances can be identified and the first three end with a false start (ca-, d-, d-, respectively). The *Mean Length of Utterance* (MLU) was calculated by dividing the total number of phonologically well-formed words by the number of utterances.

Lexical and grammatical processing. The speaker's ability to select semantically appropriate words (i.e., lexical-semantic processing) was quantified calculating a *percentage of semantic and verbal paraphasias* (e.g., Haravon et al., 1994). This was obtained by dividing the number of semantic and verbal paraphasias by the number of phonologically well-formed content words and multiplying this value by 100. Higher values represent more semantic errors per content word.

The speaker's ability to access adequate morphological and morphosyntactic information relative to the selected word (i.e., lemma level of word processing) was assessed in terms of paragrammatic errors. Accordingly, the *percentage of paragrammatic errors* was calculated by dividing the total number of paragrammatic errors by the number of phonologically well-formed words and multiplying this value by 100. Therefore higher values in this ratio in the sample represented more paragrammatic errors per word (e.g., Marini, Spoletini, et al., 2008; Marini, Tavano, et al., 2008).

The speaker's phonological skills were determined calculating a *percentage of phonological errors* (e.g., Marini, Lorusso, et al., 2007). This was derived by dividing the total number of phonological errors (i.e., false starts, phonological and phonetic paraphasias and neologisms) by the number of units and then multiplying this value by 100.

Grammatical processing was analysed in terms of percentage of complete sentences and percentage of omissions of morphosyntactic information. A sentence was considered grammatically complete if all the arguments required by a word (for example a verb) had been inserted correctly in the body of the sentence and if there were no omissions of morphosyntactic information or substitutions of free or bound morphemes. An omission of morphosyntactic information was counted each time the argument structure of a given word in a sequence was not complete. Let's consider, for example, the argumental structure required by a verb such as "hit". This word refers to an action that requires a specific morphosyntactic structure where adequate information about the agent of the action (e.g., who performs the action of hitting someone else or something) and its patient/theme (e.g., the living man or animal who experiences the action expressed by the verb, or the non-living object that receives the same action, respectively) must be correctly expressed. Therefore, a sequence such as / the man is hit by the flower-pot / is scored as a correct sentence because both agent (i.e., the flower-pot) and patient (i.e., the man) are correctly inserted in the body of the sentence. However, a sequence such as / the man is hit by . . ./ is not counted as a complete sentence because the information about the agent is missing. Therefore, in this utterance an omission of morphosyntactic information is counted. A *percentage of complete sentences* was calculated by dividing the number of grammatical sentences by the number of utterances and then multiplying this value by 100 (Saffran et al., 1989; Thompson, Shapiro, Tait, Jacobs, & Schneider, 1996). Similarly, a *percentage of omissions of morphosyntactic information* was obtained by dividing the number of omissions of morphosyntactic information by the number of utterances and then multiplying this value by 100.

Narrative organisation. As for narrative discourse organisation at the intersentential level, macro-linguistic measures included the count of errors of cohesion and of both local and global coherence relative to the utterances that form the language sample (e.g., Marini, Boewe et al., 2005; Marini, Carlomagno, et al., 2005; Marini, Spoletini, et al., 2008). Cohesiveness reflects the structural connectivity across contiguous utterances. Cohesive errors included the misuse of cohesive ties such as anaphoric pronouns, errors in number and gender agreement between pronouns or noun phrases across utterances, misuse of either cohesive function words or semantically related content words, and abrupt interruptions of utterances but at the condition that the subsequent utterances complete the previously introduced information (this kind of error has been termed *aposiopesis*; Haravon et al., 1994). As noted above, some cohesive errors can be linked to micro-linguistic processes. Consider the following sequence: / the man is staring at . . . / the man is watching the dog /. This case of self-repair exemplifies the complex relationship between micro-linguistic and macro-linguistic errors. The first utterance is incomplete because of the omission of morphosyntactic information (micro-linguistic level). However, this omission also influences the macro-linguistic organisation of the narrative. The abrupt interruption of the first utterance (scored as an occurrence of aposiopesis) causes the speaker to reformulate the sentence in the subsequent utterance(s) or to omit pieces of information that may be important for the comprehension of the story. In our example the second utterance completes the flow of thought introduced in the first one. Therefore, the abrupt interruption does not generate a local coherence error (see below). A *percentage of cohesive errors* was calculated by dividing the number of cohesive errors by the number of utterances and multiplying this value by 100.

Local coherence reflects the extent to which each utterance of the story is conceptually related to the preceding one. Local coherence errors included missing or ambiguous referents and topic switching. A topic switch occurs whenever an utterance stops abruptly (and there is a cohesive error) and the following utterance does not complete the current thought but introduces new information. For instance, in the sequence: / he's trying to. . . / these two girls are watching the dog /, the first utterance remains unfinished while the second utterance introduces new information. Missing referents are errors where the referent of a pronoun or the implicit subject of a verb (Italian is a pro-drop language) are not unambiguously clear or even incorrect. For example, consider the following sequence of utterances: / Qui stanno litigando furiosamente / Poi dice / (in English: / Here they are quarrelling furiously / Then [implicit pronoun] says /). In the second utterance there is a missing referent because it is not clear to whom the verb "dice" ("says") is referring to. The *percentage of local coherence errors* was calculated by dividing the number of local coherence errors by the number of utterances and multiplying this value by 100.

Global coherence refers to the ability to semantically relate remote utterances in the framework of a given discourse or written text. Consequently, errors of global coherence included the production of utterances that were tangential, conceptually incongruent with the story, propositional repetitions, or simply fillers (Christiansen, 1995). An utterance was considered tangential when it contained a derailment in the flow of discourse with respect to the information already provided in a preceding utterance. For instance, consider the following sequence produced during the description of the Picnic picture: / It is a picnic / I like picnics / I have made several picnics in my life /. Even though non-brain-damaged speakers often relate given facts to their own experience, in this picture description the second and the third utterances were scored as tangential, because they provided information that was irrelevant for the task and was simply triggered by a specific idea depicted in the stimulus. Therefore, while the notion of tangentiality is not always clear, in this analysis information provided by the speaker that was not directly related to events in the picture was categorised as tangential. An utterance was considered conceptually incongruent when it included ideas not directly addressed by the stimulus. Consider the following sequence produced by a speaker during the Cookie Theft picture description task: / the children are trying to get the cookies / the TV is out /. In this example the second utterance was scored as conceptually incongruent because in the picture stimulus there is no TV. A propositional repetition (see also Christiansen, 1995) was a sequence where the speaker simply repeated ideas that he/she had already provided. In these propositions, the speaker did not add any new information. Consider the following example: / the man is walking on the sidewalk / he is on the sidewalk /. In this case the second utterance simply repeats what has already been stated in the preceding one (note that a repetitive utterance does not need to contain exactly the same words of a preceding one). Finally, a filler utterance was scored whenever the speaker produced an utterance that was not providing any additional information as in the following sequence: / the man and the woman are eating / my God, and now? / ah, yes, I get it /. The last two sequences were considered as filler utterances as they reflected a moment in narration when the speaker was simply thinking about the story and what to say next. A *percentage of global coherence errors* was calculated by dividing the number of global coherence errors by the number of utterances and multiplying this value by 100 (e.g., Marini, Spoletini, et al., 2008; Marini, Boewe, et al., 2005).

Informativeness. The information content of a narrative can be evaluated at different levels. The first level refers to the production of appropriate lexical information units (LIUs), i.e., those content and function words that are not only phonologically well formed but also appropriate from a grammatical and pragmatic point of view. Therefore all those words that have been classified as semantic or verbal paraphasias, lexical fillers, lexical repetitions, paragrammatic errors, words without clear referents, or included in tangential or conceptually incongruent utterances must be excluded from the LIUs' count. A *percentage of lexical informativeness* was calculated by dividing the number of LIUs by the number of words and multiplying this value by 100. This ratio (%LIUs) has proved adequate in measuring communicative effectiveness in people with neurological or neuropsychiatric disorders—e.g., persons with right brain damage (Marini, Carlomagno, et al., 2005) or with schizophrenia (Marini, Spoletini, et al., 2008). An index of *informative speech rate* (LIUs/minute) provided additional information about the informative efficiency of the speaker. The two measures roughly correspond to functional measures of discourse production proposed by other authors. Indeed, in the CIU analysis method (Nicholas & Brookshire, 1993) the discourse efficiency is evaluated with respect to the time required to produce the narrative (Words per minute = Ws/m' and Correct Information Units per minute = CIUs/m') and extension of the sample (%CIUs = percentage of Words in the sample that are Correct Information Units). In our experience we have obtained comparable results with the two methods both with individuals with non-fluent aphasia (Marini, Caltagirone, et al., 2007) and individuals with traumatic brain injury without aphasia (e.g., Carlomagno et al., 2008).

A second way to analyse the information content of a narrative requires the identification of the thematic units contained in the language sample. A thematic unit can be defined as a main idea or detail in the story. For each of the four stimuli we have derived a series of concepts (both main ideas and details) that provide the backbone of their plots (see Marini, Carlomagno, et al., 2005, for a description of the methodology used to identify the thematic units). As a result, it becomes possible to determine how many thematic units each speaker produces with respect to all ideas that are expected to be elicited by each stimulus. The *percentage of thematic selection* for each story was calculated by dividing the number of thematic units produced in each story description by the total number of all possible thematic units for that story and multiplying this value by 100. This percentage can be considered as an index of the amount of conceptual/informational content that the speaker can derive from the eliciting stimulus (e.g., Marini, Boewe, et al., 2005; Marini, Carlomagno, et al., 2005).

TWO CASE REPORTS: AN EXAMPLE OF THE APPLICATION OF THE MULTI-LEVEL ANALYSIS OF DISCOURSE

In this section we will illustrate changes in discourse performance of two persons with different aetiologies whose linguistic recovery from severe fluent aphasia was assessed using the procedure described above. To adequately estimate the level of their impairment and subsequent recovery, this data will be presented as *z*-scores relative to a wide group of healthy participants ($N = 105$) ranging from 20 to 90 years of age. The *z*-score profile of the group of healthy participants is presented in Table 1.

TABLE 1
Z-score profile of the group of healthy participants

	Z-score						
	−3	−2	−1	0	+1	+2	+3
Words	0	3.5	43.2	82.9	122.6	162.3	202
Speech rate	25	61	97	133	169	205	241
MLU	0	2.2	4.9	7.6	10.3	13	15.7
% Phonological errors	–	–	–	0.4	1.3	2.2	3.1
% Semantic and verbal paraphasias	–	–	–	0.2	0.7	1.2	1.7
% Paragrammatic errors	–	–	–	0.3	1	1.7	2.4
% Omissions of morphosyntactic information	–	–	–	1.5	4.4	7.3	10.2
% Complete sentences	0	20.6	43.7	66.8	89.9	113	136.1
% Cohesive errors	–	–	–	2.6	7.1	11.6	16.1
% Local coherence errors	–	–	–	3.2	12	20.8	29.6
% Global coherence errors	–	–	–	1.6	6	10.4	14,8
% Lexical informativeness	63.8	72.5	81.2	89.9	98.6	107.3	116
Informative speech rate (LIUs/minute)	16.5	50	83.5	117	150.5	184	217.5
% Thematic units	10.2	28	46	63.6	81.4	99.2	117

MLU = Mean length of utterance.

MG, a medical doctor, is a 30-year-old female. In March 2003 she experienced a severe brain injury due to accidental trauma. A subdural hematoma involving the left parieto-temporal areas was confirmed by CT scan. Low attenuation changes and small subcortical haemorrhages were also evident in both hemispheres. After surgical removal of the hematoma MG slowly regained consciousness. However, she suffered from mild right hemiparesis and severe fluent aphasia. In June 2006 she was diagnosed with Wernicke's aphasia as determined by the AAT. Furthermore, the neuropsychological assessment showed the presence of subtle attention and memory deficits. She was enrolled in an intensive language stimulation programme (8 hours a week) lasting until April 2007 and focusing on word-finding difficulties and grammatical skills (e.g., completeness of sentences). In October 2006 her connected speech was assessed with the multi-level discourse analysis described earlier. This analysis was repeated in January and in April 2007, utilising a number of picture stimuli and pictures sequences (e.g., Nicholas & Brookshire, 1993) (see Table 2). An example of the language samples obtained in October 2006 is reported in the Appendix. The analysis showed slightly altered verbal productivity with an overproduction of words ($z = 2.8$), coupled with a slight reduction in MLU ($z = -1.6$) and Speech rate ($z = -1.7$). MG experienced relevant difficulties in lexical selection and some aspects of lexical access as showed by the high percentages of phonological errors ($z = 10.6$) and semantic and verbal paraphasias ($z = 4.9$). However, not all aspects of lexical processing were impaired. The almost normal production of % paragrammatic errors suggests that her ability to select and produce morphological affixes, and to coordinate the lexical and the grammatical levels of processing was quite adequate. This may seem contradictory with respect to the impaired performance in grammatical processing (% complete sentences: $z = -2.2$; % omission of morpho-syntactic information: $z = 3.5$). However, a critical inspection of her language samples (see Appendix) clearly shows that the reduced production of grammatically well-formed utterances is mainly due to the word-finding difficulties leading to frequent interruptions that made her speech quite discontinuous. This

TABLE 2
Profile of Patient MG on the three assessments performed during development of the therapeutic programme

Patient MG	*1 (October 2006)*	*2 (January 2007)*	*3 (April 2007)*
Words	2.8	2.7	3.4
Speech rate	−1.7	−1.5	−0.4
MLU	−1.6	−1.0	0.01
% Phonological errors	10.6	1.8	1.2
% Semantic and verbal paraphasias	4.9	2.4	0.0
% Paragrammatic errors	0.9	1.5	0.2
% Omissions of morphosyntactic information	3.5	1.8	−0.02
% Complete sentences	−2.2	−2.0	0.1
% Cohesive errors	13.4	10.8	3.6
% Local coherence errors	−0.1	−0.2	−0.3
% Global coherence errors	7.4	7.2	3.7
% Lexical informativeness	−4.8	−3.8	−1.4
Informative speech rate (LIUs/minute)	−2.5	−2.1	−0.7
% Thematic units	−0.7	0.17	−0.5

Values are expressed as *z*-scores with respect to normative data. MLU = Mean length of utterance.

interpretation is further confirmed by the multi-level analysis showing substantial problems in establishing cohesive ties between adjacent utterances (% cohesion errors: $z = 13.4$) and in keeping the global coherence of her narrative discourse (% global coherence errors: $z = 7.4$). Because of the many lexical and global coherence errors, MG's ability to select appropriate lexical information units was very low (% Lexical Information Units, $z = -4.8$). Therefore the multi-level analysis allowed us to have a clearer picture of her linguistic skills. During the post-therapy evaluation (April 2007, but also see the intermediate control in January 2007), the linguistic skills of MG increased. This was confirmed by her performance on the AAT. The AAT evaluation showed a generalized improvement of MG's linguistic skills: on the Token Test she did not commit any error (pre-therapy = 13), her naming performance was 114/120 (pre-therapy this test was not administrable), and on the comprehension subtest she scored 116/120 (pre-therapy 97). Furthermore, she scored 26/30 at the assessment of spontaneous language (pre-therapy not administrable). The multi-level analysis of her discourse samples confirmed the relevant changes after the treatment programme allowing us to gather more information about her narrative skills. These are illustrated in Table 2. Her lexical deficits, as indicated by the % phonological errors and % semantic and verbal paraphasias, progressively decreased to normal range. Furthermore, the reduction of word-finding difficulties led to normalisation of syntactic measures, i.e., % complete sentences ($z = 0.1$) and omission of morphosyntactic information ($z = -0.2$). This corresponded to relatively normal language informativeness (%LIUs: $z = -1.4$; LIUs/m': $z = -0.7$). Although all intrasentential measures indicated good recovery from aphasic symptoms, the analysis of the intersentential level of processing showed significant macro-linguistic deficits in establishing cohesion and global coherence (%Cohesive errors: $z = 3.6$; %Global coherence errors: $z = 3.7$). A parsimonious explanation of this last finding obviously takes into account the traumatic nature of her linguistic deficit since persons with chronic traumatic brain injury may show dissociation between recovered language processing at lexical/syntactic levels and persistent impairment at the intersentential level of discourse (Coelho, Liles, & Duffy, 1995).

Importantly, these characteristics of MG's discourse performance, highlighted by the multi-level analysis, could not be captured by a traditional standardised aphasia test.

SA was a 72-year-old male with 13 years of formal education. In 1999 he experienced left temporo-parietal ischaemia resulting in right hemianopia and severe fluent aphasia. After 12 months, in March 2000, he was diagnosed with severe Wernicke's aphasia as determined by the AAT. Because he had not received any therapy for his communicative deficit, he was enrolled in an outpatient therapy programme for persons with chronic aphasia. Pre- and post-therapy evaluation of his linguistic skills included the analysis of the language samples elicited with the picture description task in March 2000 (pre-therapy evaluation) and repeated with other standardised stimuli (e.g., Nicholas & Brookshire, 1993) at the beginning of May 2000 and at the end of June 2000 (see Table 3).

During the first interval (24 sessions in 5 weeks), SA received language stimulation therapy focusing on word-finding difficulties and production of complete sentences. In the second interval (other 24 sessions in 5 weeks), the stimulation programme in PACE format (Davis & Wilcox, 1985) focused on conveying information content of narratives in face-to-face multimodal interaction (see Carlomagno et al., 1991). The rationale for this two-step therapy programme was that he had never received language stimulation for word-finding difficulties and could take advantage from such a therapy (see Ross & Wertz, 1999; on effects of deferred language stimulation). However, given the severity of his linguistic deficit, poor response was predicted in terms of recovery of language skills. Therefore the rationale of the second treatment programme focused on the possibility that the modified PACE programme would reduce his communicative disability by stimulating multimodal communication.

The AAT evaluation after the entire therapy period failed to show any significant improvement: on the Token Test 37 errors were observed (pre-therapy = 40), naming performance was 20/120 (pre-therapy 4/120), on the comprehension subtest he scored 95/120 (pre-therapy 85). He scored 16/30 during the assessment of spontaneous language (pre-therapy = 11). However, the multi-level analysis of his discourse samples

TABLE 3

Profile of patient SA at the three evaluations: Before and after language stimulation and after modified PACE therapy (see text)

Patient SA	*1 (March, 2000)*	*2 (May 2000)*	*3 (June 2000)*
Words	−0.1	0.6	0.3
Speech rate	−3.1	−2.7	−2.4
MLU	−2	−1.8	−1.5
% Phonological errors	9.7	8.1	5.5
% Semantic and verbal paraphasias	4.5	2.5	3.0
% Paragrammatic errors	3.0	3.6	5.4
% Omissions of morphosyntactic information	3.9	3.5	2.6
% Complete sentences	−2.1	−1.6	−1.6
% Cohesive errors	10.1	9.5	6.4
% Local coherence errors	3.6	1.3	1.4
% Global coherence errors	6.1	5.3	1.2
% Lexical informativeness	−5.9	−4.9	−2.3
Informative speech rate (LIUs/minute)	−3.3	−2.9	−2.5
% Thematic units	−2.5	−2.1	−2.3

Values are expressed as *z*-scores with respect to normative data. MLU = Mean length of utterance.

showed relevant changes after each of the two treatment programmes. These are illustrated in Table 3 and will be discussed with respect to the two treatment programmes that were used.

With respect to the pre-therapy assessment (March, 2000), following the language stimulation programme very slight improvement was observed on the discourse assessment performed in May 2000. As for productivity, SA produced the same amount of words with a slight increase in speech rate (from $z=-3.1$ to $z=-2.7$) and stable MLU (from $z=-2$ to $z=-1.8$). As for his lexical processing skills, after the language stimulation programme SA produced fewer phonological errors (from $z=9.7$ to $z=8.1$) and both semantic and verbal paraphasias (from $z=4.5$ to $z=2.5$) with stable performance in the production of paragrammatic errors (from $z=3$ to $z=3.6$). Very limited improvement could be observed also on measures of syntactic accuracy (% complete sentences, from $z=-2.1$ to $z=-1.6$, and % omission of morpho-syntactic information errors, from $z=3.9$ to $z=3.5$). Therefore the limited improvement in the retrieval of lexical items did not correspond to an increase in the ability to produce grammatically complete sentences. On the functional evaluation of speech information content, this also corresponded to a persistent severe deficit in lexical informativeness (%LIUs from $z=-5.9$ to $z=-4.9$). Finally, with the exception of % Local coherence errors (from $z=3.6$ to 1.3), the other measures of intersentential organisation of narratives remained substantially unchanged (e.g., % global coherence errors from $z=6.1$ to 5.3). The results of the analysis, at the intersentential and functional level, are consistent with the chronic condition of SA's linguistic deficit. Indeed, it has been noted that people suffering from Wernicke's aphasia often show reduced pragmatic skills as their narratives contain more global coherence errors (tangential or incongruent utterances, propositional repetitions) than those produced by healthy individuals (Christiansen, 1995). The % Global coherence errors score of SA seems to confirm this hypothesis. Other changes, however, were observed on the third assessment after the development of the PACE programme. In this case, phonological errors, semantic and verbal paraphasias, and paragrammatic errors were still evident ($z=5.5$, 3.0, and 5.4, respectively). This was an expected result, as the PACE training had focused on conveying information by means of compensatory gestural behaviour. Training SA in story-telling activities, however, resulted in better skills in organising the semantic content of the stories. Global coherence errors decreased to normal range (from $z=5.3$ to 1.2) and this corresponded to increased informativeness (%LIUs from $z=-4.9$ to -2.3). This was not a surprising result. Of note, the words pertaining to tangential or semantically incongruent utterances or propositional repetitions are excluded from the %LIUs count. The reduction of these utterances in the language samples, likely due to the pragmatic component of PACE setting (Carlomagno et al., 1991; Davis & Wilcox, 1985), resulted in increased measures of speech informativeness. Therefore the multi-level procedure for discourse analysis provided useful information about the way SA used his language that could not be obtained with the simple administration of traditional aphasia tests.

CONCLUSIONS

The quantitative analysis of connected language samples from persons with brain damage is undoubtedly a time-consuming and expertise-demanding procedure. It requires time that is rarely available in the clinical routine and a good knowledge of theories of linguistic structure and processing, and of the characteristics of communicative impairment in aphasia. Nonetheless, it provides useful insight into the way these people use their language in daily-life interactions that cannot be obtained with the simple administration of traditional aphasia tests. When engaged in narrative production, speakers tend to be more fluid communicators and make use of several linguistic skills in a communicatively oriented interaction. As a consequence, the narrative analysis enables the researcher/clinician to control the interaction among several processing levels and to evaluate the communicative skills of aphasic individuals in a more ecological setting. In this sense the multi-level procedure for discourse analysis has also interesting theoretical implications, as it may provide insights on the interrelations between the different levels of linguistic processing (e.g., Prins & Bastiaanse, 2004; Sherratt, 2007).

In conclusion, the method of analysis presented in this paper has strong grounds in linguistic and psychological theories of linguistic structure and functioning. It captures several aspects of linguistic functioning providing direct information not only about a person's productivity skills and lexical and grammatical abilities, but also about his/her macro-linguistic competence and ability to select appropriate thematic and lexical information, i.e., his/her communicative and informative skills. As such, it merges both structuralist and functionalist perspectives in just one analysis.

REFERENCES

Armstrong, E. (2000). Aphasic discourse analysis: The story so far. *Aphasiology, 14*(9), 875–892.

Bates, E., Hamby, F., & Zurif, E. (1983). The effects of focal brain damage on pragmatic expression. *Canadian Journal of Psychology, 37*, 59–84.

Bloom, R. L., Borod, J. C., Santschi-Haywood, C., Pick, L. H., & Obler, L. K. (1996). Left and right hemispheric contributions to discourse coherence and cohesion. *International Journal of Neuroscience, 88*(1–2), 125–140.

Brookshire, R. H., & Nicholas, L. E. (1994). Speech sample size and test-retest stability of connected speech measures for adults with aphasia. *Journal of Speech and Hearing Research, 37*, 399–407.

Caplan, D. (1992). *Language: Structure, processing and disorders.* Cambridge, MA: MIT Press.

Carlomagno, S., Losanno, N., Emanuelli, S., & Casadio, P. (1991). Expressive language recovery or improved communicative skills: Effects of P.A.C.E. therapy on aphasics' referential communication and story retelling. *Aphasiology, 5*, 419–424.

Carlomagno, S., Giannotti, S., Vorano, L., & Marini, A. (2008). *Discourse informativeness in TBI adults without aphasic symptoms.* The 46th Annual Meeting of the Academy of Aphasia, Turku, Finland, 19–21 October 2008.

Chomsky, N. (1995). *The minimalist programme*. Cambridge, MA: MIT Press.

Christiansen, J. A. (1995). Coherence violations and propositional usage in the narratives of fluent aphasics. *Brain and Language, 51*, 291–317.

Coelho, C. A., Liles, B. Z., & Duffy, R. J. (1995). Impairments of discourse abilities and executive functions in traumatically brain-injured adults. *Brain Injury, 9*(5), 471–477.

Davis, G., O'Neil-Pirozzi, T., & Coon, M. (1997). Referential cohesion and logical coherence of narration after right hemisphere stroke. *Brain and Language, 56*, 183–210.

Davis, G., & Wilcox, M. (1985). *Adult aphasia rehabilitation: Applied pragmatics.* Windsor, UK: NFER-Nelson.

Doyle, P. J., Goda, A. J., & Spencer, K. A. (1995). The communicative informativeness and efficiency of connected discourse by adults with aphasia under structured and conversational sampling conditions. *American Journal of Speech-Language Pathology, 4*, 130–134.

Easterbrook, A., Byers Brown, A., & Perera, K. (1982). A comparison of speech of adult aphasic subjects in spontaneous and structured interaction. *International Journal of Language and Communication Disorders, 17*(3), 93–107.

Frederiksen, C. H., Bracewell, R. J., Breuleux, A., & Renaud, A. (1990). The cognitive representation and processing of discourse: Function and dysfunction. In Y. Joanette & H. Brownell (Eds.), *Discourse ability and brain damage: Theoretical and empirical perspectives*. New York: Springer Verlag.

Garrett, M. F. (1980). Levels of processing in sentence production. In B. Butterworth (Ed.), *Language production: Speech and talk* (Vol. 1, pp. 177–220), London: Academic Press.

Glosser, G., & Deser, T. (1990). Patterns of discourse production among neurological patients with fluent language disorders. *Brain and Language, 40*(1), 67–88.

Goodglass, H., & Kaplan, E. (1972). *The Boston Diagnostic Aphasia Examination*. Philadelphia, PA: Lea & Febiger.

Grice, H. P. (1975). Logic and conversation. In P. Cole & J. P. Morgan (Eds.), *Syntax and semantics: Speech acts* (pp. 41–58). New York: Academic Press.

Halliday, M. A. K., & Hasan, R. (1976). *Cohesion in English*. London: Longman.

Haravon, A., Obler, L., & Sarno, M. (1994). A method for microanalysis of discourse in brain-damaged patients. In R. Bloom, L. Obler, S. De Santi, & J. Ehrlich (Eds.), *Discourse analysis and applications: Studies in adult clinical populations* (pp. 47–80). Hillsdale, NJ: Lawrence Erlbaum Associates Inc.

Helm-Estabrooks, N. A., Fitzpatrick, P. M., & Barresi, B. (1981). Response of an agrammatic patient to a syntax stimulation programme for aphasia. *Journal of Speech and Hearing Disorders, 46*, 422–427.

Helm-Estabrooks, N. A., & Ramsberger, G. (1986). Treatment of agrammatism in long-term Broca's aphasia. *British Journal of Disorders of Communication, 21*(1), 39–45.

Huber, W., & Gleber, J. (1982). Linguistic and non-linguistic processing of narratives in aphasia. *Brain and Language, 16*, 1–18.

Indefrey, P., & Levelt, W. J. M. (2000). The neural correlates of language production. In M. S. Gazzaniga (Ed.), *The new cognitive neurosciences* (2nd ed., pp. 845–865). Cambridge, MA: MIT Press.

Indefrey, P., & Levelt, W. J. M. (2004), The spatial and temporal signatures of word production components. *Cognition*, 92, 101–144.

Jakobs, B. J. (2001). Social validity of changes in informativeness and efficiency of aphasic discourse following linguistic specific treatment (LST). *Brain and Language, 78*, 115–127.

Jakobson, R. (1980). On aphasic disorders from a linguistic angle. In R. Jakobson (Ed.), *The framework of language*. Ann Arbor, MI: University of Michigan Press.

Johnson-Laird, P. N. (1980). Mental models in cognitive science. *Cognitive Science, 4*, 71–115.

Kertesz, A. (1982). *Western Aphasia Battery*. New York: Grune & Stratton

Kintsch, W. (1994). Text comprehension, memory, and learning. *American Psychologist, 49*, 294–303.

Kintsch, W., & Van Dijk, T. (1978). Toward a model of text comprehension and production. *Psychological Review, 85*, 363–394.

Larfeuil, C., & Le Dorze, G. (1997). An analysis of the word-finding difficulties and of the content of the discourse of recent and chronic aphasic speakers. *Aphasiology, 11*(8), 783–811.

Levelt, W. J. M. (1989). *Speaking: from intention to articulation*. Cambridge, MA: MIT Press.

Levelt, W. J. M., Roelofs, A., & Meyer, A. S. (1999). A theory of lexical access in speech production. *Behavioral and Brain Sciences, 22*, 1–38.

Levinson, S. C. (1983). *Pragmatics*. Cambridge, UK: Cambridge University Press.

Luzzatti, C., Willems, K., & DeBleser, R. (1991). *Aachener Aphasie Test (Versione Italiana)*. Firenze, Italy: Organizzazioni Speciali.

Marini, A., Boewe, A., Caltagirone, C., & Carlomagno, S. (2005). Age-related differences in the production of textual descriptions. *Journal of Psycholinguistic Research, 34*(5), 439–463.

Marini, A., Caltagirone, C., Pasqualetti, P., & Carlomagno, S. (2007). Patterns of language improvement in adults with non-chronic non-fluent aphasia after specific therapies. *Aphasiology, 21*(2), 164–186.

Marini A., Carlomagno S., Caltagirone C., & Nocentini U. (2005) The role played by the right hemisphere in the organisation of complex textual structures. *Brain and Language, 93*(1), 46–54.

Marini, A., Lorusso, M. L., D'Angelo, G., Civati, F., Turconi, A.C., Fabbro, F., et al. (2007). Evaluation of narrative abilities in patients suffering from Duchenne Muscular Dystrophy. *Brain and Language*, *102*(1), 1–12.

Marini, A., Martelli, S., Gagliardi, C., Fabbro, F., & Borgatti, R. (2010). Narrative language in Williams' syndrome and its neuropsychological correlates. *Journal of Neurolinguistics*, *23*, 97–111.

Marini, A., Spoletini, I., Rubino, I. A., Ciuffa, M., Bria, P., Martinotti, G., et al. (2008). The language of schizophrenia: An analysis of micro and macro-linguistic abilities and their neuropsychological correlates. *Schizophrenia Research*, *105*, 144–155.

Marini, A., Tavano, A., & Fabbro, F. (2008). Assessment of linguistic abilities in Italian children with specific language impairment. *Neuropsychologia*, *46*, 2816–2823.

Mayer, J. F., & Murray, L. (2003). Functional measures of naming in aphasia: Word retrieval in confrontation naming versus connected speech. *Aphasiology*, *17*, 481–497.

Nicholas, L., & Brookshire, R. (1993). A system for quantifying the informativeness and efficiency of the connected speech of adults with aphasia. *Journal of Speech Hearing Research*, *36*(2), 338–350.

Oelschlaeger, M. L., & Thorne, J. C. (2000). Application of the Correct Information Units Analysis to the naturally occurring conversation of a person with aphasia. *Journal of Speech, Language and Hearing Research*, *42*, 636–648.

Olness, G. S., Matteson, S. E., & Stewart, C. T. (2010). "Let me tell you the point": How speakers with aphasia assign prominence to information in narratives. *Aphasiology*, *24*(6–8), 697–708.

Prins, R., & Bastiaanse, R. (2004). Analysing the spontaneous speech of aphasic patients. *Aphasiology*, *18*(12), 1075–1091.

Prins, R. S., Snow, C. E., & Wagenaar, E. (1978). Recovery from aphasia: Spontaneous speech versus language comprehension. *Brain and Language*, *6*, 192–211.

Rochon, E., Saffran, E. M., Berndt, R. S., & Schwartz, M. F. (2000). Quantitative analysis of aphasic sentence production: Further development and new data. *Brain and Language*, *72*, 193–218.

Ross, K. B., & Wertz, R. (1999). Comparison of impairment and disability measures for assessing severity of, and improvement in, aphasia. *Aphasiology*, *13*, 113–124.

Saffran, E. M., Berndt, R. S., & Schwartz, M. F. (1989). The quantitative analysis of agrammatic production: Procedure and data. *Brain and Language*, *37*, 440–479.

Schwartz, M. F., Saffran, E. M., Fink, R. B., Myers, J. L., & Martin, N. (1994). Mapping therapy: A treatment programme for agrammatism. *Aphasiology*, *8*, 19–54.

Sherratt, S. (2007). Multi-level discourse analysis: A feasible approach. *Aphasiology*, *21*(3/4), 375–393.

Shewan, C. M. (1988). The Shewan Spontaneous Language Analysis (SSLA) system for aphasic adults: Description, reliability and validity. *Journal of Communication Disorders*, *21*, 103–138.

Sperber, D., & Wilson, D. (1986). *Relevance. Communication and cognition*. Oxford, UK: Blackwell.

Springer, L., Huber, W., Schlenck, K. J., & Schlenck, C. (2000). Agrammatism: Deficit or compensation? Consequences for aphasia therapy. *Neuropsychological Rehabilitation*, *10*(3), 279–309.

Thompson, C. K., Shapiro, L. P., Tait, M., Jacobs, B., & Schneider, S. L. (1996). Training wh-question production in agrammatic aphasia: Analysis of argument and adjunct movement. *Brain and Language*, *52*, 175–228.

Ulatowska, H. K., Freedman-Stern, R., Doyel, A. W., Macaluso-Haynes, S., & North, A. J. (1983). Production of narrative discourse in aphasia. *Brain and Language*, *19*(2), 317–334.

Ulatowska, H. K., North, A. J., & Macaluso-Hayes, S. (1981). Production of narrative discourse and procedural discourse in aphasia. *Brain and Language*, *13*(2), 345–371.

Van Leer, E., & Turkstra, L. (1999). The effect of elicitation task on discourse coherence and cohesion in adolescents with brain injury. *Journal of Communication Disorders*, *32*(5), 327–348.

Vermeulen, J., Bastiaanse, R., & van Wageningen, B. (1989). Spontaneous speech in aphasia: A correlational study. *Brain and Language*, *36*, 252–274.

Wagenaar, E., Snow, C., & Prins, R.S. (1975). Spontaneous speech of aphasic patients: A psycholinguistic analysis. *Brain and Language*, *2*, 281–303.

Yorkston, K. M., & Beukelman, D. R. (1980). An analysis of connected speech samples of aphasic and normal speakers. *Journal of Speech and Hearing Disorders*, *45*, 27–36.

APPENDIX

Patient MG

Vaso in testa (ottobre 2006)	Flower pot (October 2006)
/ Qui abbiamo il primo momento in cui il signore che ha l . . . / cane / trova / anzi viene colpito in testa dalla . . . / dal . . . / dalla [p:one] / non so come si possa chiamare / comunque da quel pane che gli è caduto giù dalla / . . . terrazza /. . . . sopra / e lui si arrabbia / e inizia a contestare / a dir un sacco di parole contro il signore che ha / che è il signore della . . . / cosa / e quindi delle / . . . ferra / delle . . . / [ferrate] come quella insomma / e è arrabbiato / inizia a dargliene / a dirgliene qua. / alcune contro il vesti / vestibolo / e si arrabbia talmente tanto che prende il cane e ritorna ad andare . . . / di . . . / trovare il signore che consce / che adesso conosce . . . / a bussare alla . . . / po / porta / dopo un po' esce una signora con un carro / e è molt / molto gentile / e infatti già sorridendo si / . . . a- / adopera verso il . . . / bess / bessotto / bessotto / forse un bassotto / e lo aiuta / il signore / il maschio che fino a quel momento è rimasto a prendersele le posate da lei si ferma a . . . / baciale la / la . . . / mano / e intanto il suo . . . / cane se ne va con la / con la . . . / la . . . / somma / con il . . . / il . . . / la . . . / l'altra [cherpa] che aveva preso in va . . . / in . . . / nella . . . / bocca del . . . / del vivaio /	/ Here we have the first moment when the man who has f- / dog / finds / well, is hit on his head from the . . . / from the . . . / from the [p:one] / I don't know how to say this / anyway, from that bread that has fallen down from the . . . / balcony / . . . above . . . / and he get angry / and begins to protest / to say many words against the man who has / who is the man of the . . . / thing / and so of the . . . / ir- / of the . . . / [ironates] like that, well / and he is angry / he starts giving them to her / saying to her th- / some against the ha- / hallway / and he gets so much angry that he takes his dog and comes back to go . . . / to . . . / find the man whom he kn- / whom he now knows / to knock at the . . . / d- / door / after a while a lady comes out with a wagon / and she is ver- / very nice / indeed already smiling he / b- / bends to the sau- / sausage deg / sausage deg / perhaps a sausage dog / and helps him / the man / the male who until that moment has been waiting to get to him the cutlery from her stops to . . . / kiss her the / the . . . / hand / in the meanwhile the . . . / dog goes away with the / with the . . . / the . . . / sum / with the . . . / the . . . / the . . . / the other [cherpa] that had taken in va- . . . / in . . . / in the . . . / mouth of the . . . / of the nursery /

An example of narrative produced by MG. The story has been elicited in 169 seconds and was made of 222 units, and 60 utterances. A total of 7.7 % of the units were phonological errors (9 false starts, 4 phonological paraphasias and 4 neologisms). Consequently, she produced 205 phonologically well-formed words with a speech rate of 72.8 words per minute with a MLU of 3.4 words per utterance. Of the 205 words, 8 were semantic paraphasias (3.9%) and 1 was a paragrammatic error (0.5%). Furthermore, of the 60 utterances produced, 25 presented with omissions of morphosyntactic information (12.2%) and barely 8 of them were complete sentences (13.3%). When analysing her macrolinguistic skills, we found that the description is filled with utterance interruptions, as 36 of the 60 utterances produced were abruptly interrupted (% Cohesive errors: 60%). However, only 1 word had missing referent and no topic shift was detected (%Local coherence errors: 3.3%). Furthermore, 1 utterance was a filler sentence, 11 were propositional repetitions, 2 were conceptually incongruent with the story, and 1 was tangential. Consequently, 25% of the utterances were violations of global coherence. Furthermore, on the functional analysis of MG's description, several problems in lexical informativeness can be detected. Only 90 of the 205 words produced in this description were lexical information units

(%LIU = 43.9%). Indeed, besides the lexical and morphological errors, the patient produced 23 lexical fillers, 48 lexical repetitions, 1 passe-par-tout, 11 words included in propositional repetitions, 18 in conceptually incongruent utterances, and 4 in tangential sequences. Furthermore, she produced LIUs at a rate of 32 LIUs per minute. Finally the analysis showed that she produced 54% of expected thematic units, therefore suggesting normal to near-normal ability to select appropriate concepts about the story.

APHASIOLOGY, 2011, 25 (11), 1393–1413

Personal narratives in aphasia: Coherence in the context of use

Gloria Streit Olness[1] and Hanna K. Ulatowska[2]

[1]University of North Texas, Denton, TX, USA
[2]University of Texas at Dallas, Dallas, TX, USA

Background: Discourse functionality is a primary goal of aphasia assessment and intervention. People who have aphasia often display a paradoxical functionality in their production of discourse, despite their aphasic impairment. A variety of linguistic and non-linguistic resources are orchestrated to produce coherent discourse. One discourse genre, the *personal story*, is ubiquitous and fills important intrapersonal and interpersonal functions.

Aims: The primary objective is to provide a framework for the structure and function of personal stories, to guide future clinical discourse research towards development of practical clinical assessment of discourse functionality in people who have aphasia.

Main Contribution: Characteristics of personal stories in their context of use are discussed for their contributions to overall discourse coherence. Examples of coherent and incoherent personal stories narrated by people who have aphasia illustrate interactions among coherence-building resources. The influence of group contexts and cultural contexts on coherence of personal stories is considered.

Conclusions: It is the interaction, and not the componential addition, of multiple resources that supports coherent production of personal stories in context. Qualitative frameworks need to be integrated with quantitative approaches as we develop reliable and valid means of functional discourse assessment. An understanding of the lives of people who have aphasia will be essential for defining the most meaningful and functional contexts for our discourse assessments.

Keywords: Aphasia; Personal narratives; Functional assessment; Coherence.

Functional communication is the metaphorical holy grail of rehabilitation outcomes in aphasia intervention. Elman and Bernstein-Ellis (1995) note that the term *functional* has been used traditionally by the field to highlight the importance of communicating via any means possible, as related to the use of compensatory strategies; and to emphasise the importance of choosing activities and tasks that are relevant to individual clients. Others have defined functional improvements to be those that generalise to settings other than the clinic (e.g., Garrett & Pimentel, 2007). Whether one takes an impairment-based approach to treatment, a psychosocial approach to treatment, or some combination of both, the primary goal of assessment is to characterise a client's

Address correspondence to: Gloria Streit Olness, University of North Texas, Department of Speech and Hearing Sciences, 1155 Union Circle # 305010, Denton, Texas 76203-5017, USA. E-mail: golness@unt.edu

Our sincere thanks to the participant volunteers who take part in our research. We extend our appreciation to two anonymous reviewers for their helpful and insightful comments. A portion of the discourse samples presented here was collected with the support of a grant from the NIH/NIDCD (1R03DC005151-01) awarded to the first author.

http://dx.doi.org/10.1080/02687038.2011.599365

(capacity for) communicative competence, and the ultimate therapeutic goal for the client with aphasia is functional communication.

One result of this focus on functionality has been an emphasis on the ecological validity of our assessment and treatment contexts. Tasks and activities are specifically chosen to represent *daily contexts* of communication that are *naturalistic* or *realistic* (Elman & Bernstein-Ellis, 1995), such as script training (Cherney, Halper, Holland & Cole, 2008). Driven by similar motivations to assess in naturalistic contexts, many clinical researchers have analysed discourse under the premise that discourse is the manifestation of language in its very context of use (e.g., Cherney, Shadden & Coelho, 1998).

While the goal in discourse aphasiology has been to gather samples representative of *functional* communication, Armstrong (2000) comments that many analyses of discourse have focused on *structural* microlinguistic phenomena, such as lexical and syntactic phenomena, uninterpreted for their influence on overall discourse function. Based on clinical observations, one might surmise that the influence of microstructure on discourse functionality may be limited. Audrey Holland has highlighted the ability of aphasic persons to "communicate better than they talk" (1977, p. 173) and has commented that there is little relationship between severity of language impairment and the ability to cope and function in daily life (Holland, 2010). As an example, in one aphasia group familiar to the first author, a group member with limited verbal output and no augmentative device told humorous life stories that were so funny that group members laughed to the point of tears. Likewise, Sacks (2010) describes a woman with severe aphasia who resumed an active and communicative social life, despite little change in her underlying impairment.

To help account for this enigmatic functionality, our clinical discourse research should address the variety of linguistic/paralinguistic resources (e.g., lexicon, morphosyntax, prosody) and non-linguistic resources (e.g., shared world knowledge of culturally predictable patterns of discourse structure; knowledge of the cultural and interpersonal context) as they are *orchestrated together* by aphasic communicators to communicate coherently (Ulatowska & Olness, 2007). It is also important to consider the contexts in which these resources and strategies are successfully tapped, as tools for social meaning making (Armstrong & Ferguson, 2010). Finally, whatever the means of sampling and analysing discourse, clinical researchers should scrutinise the ecological validity of their research designs by explicitly addressing the way in which their sampling and analysis reflects functional use of discourse in naturalistic contexts.

At the same time, a complete picture of communicative competence should also outline limitations or boundaries on this competence, perhaps based in part on the underlying impairment, and the contexts in which these boundaries are manifested. For example, in a recent court case a woman with aphasia who had been assaulted was capable of telling her family, her care team, and the police what happened. However, in the context of a legal competency hearing in which she was not allowed rightful accommodations, she was initially deemed incompetent to testify in her case (National Aphasia Association and W. Murphy, personal communication). Likewise, there is evidence to suggest that when speakers with aphasia are telling personal narratives in monologue, the normally preserved ability to make a "point" with a personal story may be compromised if the aphasic impairment is too severe (Olness, Matteson, & Stewart, 2010).

The current paper will attempt to provide a partial framework to guide future discourse research, geared towards development of practical clinical approaches to assessment of *communicative competence* or *functionality* of persons with aphasia. In the past, one of the roadblocks to analysis of discourse in the clinic has been the perception that sampling and analysis need to be labour intensive. However, the roadblock of transcription may be circumvented if, as a field, we can build a solid, shared understanding of the primary functions of personal narratives and how these functions are filled, and if on-line criterion-referenced and behavioural observations of spontaneous storytelling can be designed based on this understanding. Ultimately, clinically efficient, feasible, and valid screening and assessment in the form of transcription-less discourse-based analysis may be possible, supported by future studies of the degree to which qualitative approaches are reliable, sensitive to change over time (cf. Armstrong, 1997), and externally valid relative to quantitative, transcription-based discourse measures (cf. Armstrong, Brady, Mackenzie, & Norrie, 2007).

Discussion will focus specifically on one ubiquitous discourse type, namely *personal narrative* or *story*. A focus on one particular discourse genre is consistent with the suggestion by Armstrong (2000) that mixing samples from different genres may be problematic for analysis and interpretation.

In a fashion analogous to American models of evidence-based practice (Dollaghan, 2007), these clinical assessment suggestions will be derived from more than one source: basic research and discourse models; clinical expertise; insights of clients with aphasia and their family, friends, and peers; and data-based examples from research and the clinic. The authors will not attempt to be comprehensive in coverage of the clinical discourse literature as a whole; rather the goal is to be coherent in discussion of the frameworks and evidence that are relevant for assessing aphasic clients' functional use of personal narratives in particular.

BACKGROUND

Scope of discussion

Theoretical and clinical discussion in the current paper will concentrate on production of one sub-type of the *narrative* genre of discourse, namely *personal stories*, which will also be interchangeably referenced in the current paper as *personal narratives*. Consistent with the focus on story production, discussion in the current paper will place relatively less emphasis on the following: production of narratives that are not personal narratives, such as narrative productions in response to pictures or prompts for pre-set story retells; comprehension of narratives; and production and comprehension of other discourse genres such as procedural and expository discourse (Longacre, 1996). These topics will be considered only to the degree that they may shed light on the targeted discussion of the personal story production.

Motivations for assessment of personal narratives

Narrative research, direct observations and self-reflection attest to the ubiquity of personal stories in daily contexts of communication. Labov (1997) comments that "narratives are privileged forms of discourse that play a central role in almost every conversation" (p. 396). Narratives are so pervasive in the daily life of *Homo narrans* that researchers have used conversational telling of personal narratives to explore cultural values and assumptions (e.g., Johnstone, 1990; Polanyi, 1989) and to create historical cultural archives (StoryCorps, 2010). Moreover, systematic rules for incorporation of narratives into conversation have been extensively described (Ervin-Tripp & Küntay, 1996; Norrick, 2000; Schegloff, 1982). One would be hard-pressed to encounter a typical day in which personal stories are not told or heard, whether these are short stories of a few sentences such as an account of a near collision on the highway that day, or longer stories of a salient turning point in one's life, such as the story of one's stroke.

Even more importantly, personal stories are *multi-functional*. Narrative proper fills two basic functions: referential and evaluative (cf. Jakobson, 1990). Polanyi (1989) states that a narrator's two primary tasks are to give enough detail to events to state the events clearly (referential function) and to highlight the important information in the narrative to add salience to it (evaluative function). In its referential function, narrative *refers* to the *who*, *what*, *when*, *where*, and *what happened* of the narrated event (Labov, 1972). In its evaluative function, narrative *evaluates* the speaker's attitude and opinions about the event, i.e., the *so what* of the narrated event or why the story was told in the first place (Labov, 1972). Of these two functions, the evaluative function may be the key function associated with storytelling. Polanyi (1989) comments that the primary reason that a story is told is not to convey the sequence of events proper, but rather "to make a point, to transmit a message—often some sort of moral evaluation or implied critical judgment—about the world the teller shares with other people" (p. 16). Research evidence suggests that the narrative referential function is particularly vulnerable in narrators who have aphasia (Ulatowska, Allard, & Chapman, 1990). However, the primary evaluative function may be spared overall, unless the aphasic impairment and associated referential problems are relatively severe (Armstrong & Ulatowska, 2007; Olness & Englebretson, 2011; Olness et al., 2010).

Based largely on their evaluative potential, narratives also fill intrapersonal and interpersonal functions. At the intrapersonal level, tellings and retellings of personal stories allow the narrator to "relive, re-evaluate and reconstruct remembered experience" (Norrick, 2000, p. 2). Across a lifetime, such *storying* and *re-storying* through life review and reminiscence is part of *biographical ageing*, associated with reinterpretation of life events as they relate to one's life as a whole, and ultimately manifesting one's *ordinary wisdom* (Kenyon, 2006; Randall & Kenyon, 2001). At the interpersonal level, shared stories also provide a way to present oneself and one's identity to others, and to bond through shared experience and shared culture (e.g., Johnstone, 1990).

Notably, the need to accomplish the intrapersonal and interpersonal functions associated with narratives remains, whether or not the narrator has aphasia. To the degree that aphasia affects the ability to tell personal stories, it may also affect the ability to accomplish these narrative functions. The sharing of illness narratives in particular is a way to cope with the impairment and its impact on one's identity and life goals (Frank, 1997; Kleinman, 1988). As Frank (1997, p. 1) notes, "(s)erious illness is a loss of the 'destination and map' that had previously guided the ill person's life: ill people have to learn 'to think differently.' They learn by hearing themselves tell their stories, absorbing others' reactions, and experiencing their stories being shared".

It is a bitter irony that people who have aphasia have diminished ability to tell their stories, at the very time when they need to tell them. Shadden (2005) speaks of the "theft" of one's identity that is associated with the onset of aphasia. Following stroke, the importance of exchange of personal stories in the setting of an aphasia group cannot be underestimated as a way to assist group members in "re-creating their own identities and future selves" (Bernstein-Ellis & Elman, 2007, p. 76). As Holland (2007) notes, the opportunity for clients with aphasia to exchange stories of their strokes and stroke aftermath, in particular, has healing power. Indeed it is selective self-disclosure of one's attitudes and feelings, such as expressed through personal narratives (Armstrong & Ulatowska, 2007), that is hypothesised to be the key factor for people in crisis to reap benefits from group membership (Ewing, 2007). A promising basis for future research on the functions of shared personal stories for people with aphasia, such as stories of stroke, has emerged with the advent of shared multimedia databases of personal stories (AphasiaBank, 2011; Aphasia Corner Blog, 2011; StoryCorps, 2010). These have also created venues outside of aphasia group settings for people to share their personal stories of life with aphasia.

Discourse coherence as a basis for communicative competence

For a person with aphasia to be communicatively competent and functional in their expression of discourse, the discourse needs to be coherent. This relationship between communicative competence and discourse coherence is the working assumption under which the current paper operates. A discourse is defined as coherent when it "hangs together" or makes sense as a whole, in its context of use (Ulatowska & Olness, 2004).

The construct of coherence as defined here is related to the notion of *global coherence* as defined by Glosser (1993), which is the overall semantic unity of themes and topics in a discourse. However, the two are different in how they are operationalised. Global coherence is operationalised by Glosser through a series of ratings of the contributions of the semantic content of *each individual sentence within the text* to the semantic unity of the discourse as a whole. In contrast, coherence as defined in the current paper can be operationalised only through a single rating of the semantic unity of the whole discourse-situated-in-context, i.e., the degree to which this unit, as a whole, hangs together or makes sense.

The current paper further assumes that coherence is achieved through the integration of multiple semantic resources, e.g., information expressed in the text through a variety of linguistic and paralinguistic tools; knowledge of the world and the predictable ways in which discourse is structured; and the relevant characteristics of the context in which the discourse is being produced. Correspondingly, linguistic competence does not necessarily predict communicative competence. Rather it is how well speakers with aphasia integrate the meanings created by the linguistic and paralinguistic resources they have at hand, with their understanding of the world and the way discourse is structured in their culture, while remaining sensitive to the relevant features of the context in which they are communicating, to achieve targeted functions (cf. Saville-Troike, 2003). These functions include both the referential function of narratives and the evaluative function, which entail coherence of both referential and evaluative content. In sum, language is one set of meaning-making resources (Armstrong & Ferguson, 2010) that combines with other resources to achieve communicative functions through discourse.

The following section discusses some of the key resources that contribute to coherent production of narrative discourse. This will be followed by a qualitative assessment of both coherent and incoherent personal stories of speakers with aphasia, to illustrate the ways in which various linguistic forms and predictable discourse structures function together to create coherence, with the assumption that use of the forms and structures is driven by their function. Following Saville-Troike (2003, p. 14), this assumption of "(the) primacy of function over form in analysis is not to deny or neglect the formal structures of communication; rather it is to require integration of function and form in analysis and description."

THE PREDICTABLE NATURE OF NARRATIVE

Narratives as a discourse genre, and personal stories as a subtype of that genre, have certain prototypical characteristics. This culturally shared knowledge about the nature of narratives contributes to the overall coherence of personal stories by bolstering both coherence of referential content and coherence of evaluative content. To the degree that these culturally shared characteristics of narrative are effectively combined in a personal story, the story will meet audience expectations for the means by which stories fill their referential and evaluative functions, thus increasing the story's coherence. Special note should be made that not all of these characteristics make high demands on linguistic competence, which may assist storytellers with aphasia to produce coherent stories despite their linguistic impairment. It is this very possibility of narrative coherence in the face of linguistic impairment that is explored in the current work.

Narrative superstructure

An overarching pattern in narratives that contributes to overall coherence of personal stories is the narrative superstructure (van Dijk & Kintsch, 1983), also referenced as the story schema (Mandler, 1984). Key components of the superstructure, in rough sequential order, are the orientation or setting, initiating event, complicating action, result or resolution, and coda (Berman, 1997; Labov, 1972). In general terms, one may refer to the "beginning, middle, and end" of a story. The canonical ordering of superstructure is relatively preserved in aphasia, although exceptions may occur in speakers with relatively more severe aphasia. Overall, this predictable pattern enhances the overall coherence of personal stories told by aphasic narrators. Referential and evaluative content are conveyed in and through narrative superstructure in predictable ways that are detailed below.

Narrative characteristics that support the referential function

Narratives make reference to person, action, time, and location. The referential function, i.e., expression of the *who*, *what*, *when*, *where*, and *what happened* (Labov, 1972), may be particularly vulnerable in narrators who have aphasia (Ulatowska et al., 1990); overall clarity of reference may be reduced largely as a consequence of the anomia which defines the very nature of the disorder. The verb in particular has been recognised to play an important role at the level of the sentence, and studies suggest that the verb, which references activity, may be compromised at the word and sentence levels among individuals who have aphasia (e.g., Bastiaanse & Zonneveld, 1998; Edwards & Bastiaanse, 1998).

Reference has been explored in aphasia largely through the construct of cohesion. Discourse cohesion is achieved through the use of "the set of possibilities that exist *in the language* for making text hang together [as a larger unit]" (Halliday & Hasan, 1976, p. 18; emphasis added, to differentiate cohesion from the semantic notion of coherence). The notion of cohesion encompasses not only lexical reference but also conjunction and ellipsis, which together create systems of anaphoric and cataphoric linkages which coalesce to make text cohesive. Problems with narrative cohesion in aphasia may well be associated with overall reductions in narrative coherence (Armstrong, 2000).

It is the contention of the current paper that problems with the referential function and associated cohesion pose the primary threat to coherence of personal narratives for speakers with aphasia, and it is only through the use of other coherence-building resources that narrators with aphasia are so often able to produce coherent personal stories. For example, both Ulatowska et al. (1990) and Glosser and Deser (1990) suggest that discourse coherence is possible despite significant difficulties at the lexical and sentential levels. Christiansen (1995) and Huber (1990) highlight contrasting examples in which difficulties with lower linguistic levels ultimately do seem to impact discourse coherence. The challenge for researchers and clinicians is to tease apart the factors that play a role in such inconsistencies, in a way that can be applied to clinical practice.

Characteristics of personal stories associated with the referential function are: focus on agents and their activities, a linear temporal-causal organisation of narrative events set in past time, and inclusion of key background information.

Focus on agents and their activities. Reference to specific agents and their activities is a key characteristic of personal narratives, as contrasted with other genres of discourse such as procedural or expository discourse (Longacre, 1996). What have been relatively unexplored in the clinical discourse literature, to our knowledge, are the relative effects of poor reference to key story agents and their activities, versus ancillary story agents and their activities, since not all agents in a story can be presumed to carry equal cohesive weight.

Linear temporal-causal organisation. Narratives are structured with a temporal-causal "backbone" of narrative clauses or utterances, termed the *narrative event line*, that corresponds with the order of happenings in the narrated event (Berman, 1997; Labov, 1972; Labov & Waletzky, 1967; Longacre, 1996), e.g., *This boy punched me; And I punched him; And the teacher came in; And (she) stopped the fight.* (Labov, 1972, p. 360). As noted by Polanyi (1989), a narrative "models the passage of time in some world by building up a time line demarcated by discrete moments at which instantaneous occurrences are reported to take place" (p. 16). Use of this predictable ordering enhances the coherence of a personal narrative. The narrative event line typically starts with the initiating event of the narrative superstructure, and extends through the complicating action and resolution (Berman, 1997).

The temporal-referential ability to sequence one's narrative utterances to represent the order of the narrated events *is not dependent on any lexical or syntactic abilities* per se; temporal-causal markers like *then* or *so* need not be expressed, and utterances need only be put in their correct sequence. For this reason the presence of aphasia does not necessarily affect one's ability to use temporal-causal order in personal narratives. Thus temporal-causal ordering of utterances may be a key contributor to the coherence of stories told by people with aphasia, even though there may be a potential shortening of the temporal-causal event line in aphasia (Ulatowska, Olness, & Williams, 2004), especially in cases of more severe aphasia (Olness, 2006).

Utterances on the narrative event line often include distinctive verb content, verb tense-aspect morphology, and adverbials (e.g., *all of a sudden*) that redundantly highlight the punctiliar nature of the event sequence (Olness, 2006). However, it is not clear that verbs and verb morphology are absolutely necessary to represent the event sequence, so this factor may not affect the ability of aphasic narrators to establish a narrative event line. Explicit linguistic marking is needed only when the story diverges from this order, as in a flashback. On the other hand, a different combination of aspect and modality markings are found in those utterances that are off the event line, i.e., those containing background and evaluative information (Olness, 2006). Thus the verb system may be important for differentiating narrative information that is on the event line from information that is off the event line.

Events set in past time. Another key referential characteristic of personal stories, related to temporal reference in particular, is that personal stories provide an account of events that occurred in the past (Longacre, 1996). Thus past tense markings will be found on verbs throughout the narrative. However, even when agrammatism or paragrammatism affects the use of past tense morphology in the personal narrative of a speaker with aphasia, temporal reference is unlikely to be negatively affected. The reason is that the events represented in personal narratives are presumed a priori to have occurred in the past, so the use of past tense morphology is a redundant marker. In conversation, the shift back to the "here and now" typically occurs only after the story is complete, with a shift to present tense in the story's coda (Labov, 1972), e.g., *That's it.*

On the other hand, even though stories are set in the past tense, differential use of non-past tense and a variety in aspect markings may appear in the use of *direct speech*, i.e., direct quotes of narrative characters (Ulatowska & Olness, 2001; Ulatowska, Olness, Wertz, & Hill, 2002). For example, present tense and perfective aspect of African American Vernacular English (AAVE) are used in a quote within a stroke story: "*It kinda look* (PRES) *like she done* (PERF) *had a stroke*" (Ulatowska, 2010, p. 139). Thus some facility with verbs and verb morphology may contribute to overall coherence.

Inclusion of background information. Production of personal stories assumes the inclusion of background informative or descriptive elements which "take into account what the addressee might want to know or needs to know" (Berman, 1997, p. 241). For example, *We kids were at school one day. I was ten at the time and this other kid was thirteen* might be given as background information in the story of an attack by a school bully. This background information is important for making a personal story coherent. It is typically concentrated in the setting portion of the superstructure, but can be found in other structural components of the narrative as well (Berman, 1997).

Certainly the reference problems associated with aphasia may impact the clarity of this background information, and thus impact the overall coherence of the story. On the other hand, much background information is culturally shared and predictable, e.g., script knowledge (Schank & Abelson, 1977), which reduces the demands on the referential system. So, for example, once the narrator has established that the setting of the story is a school, other referential details about the usual school routine can be omitted. Shared cultural knowledge may be one of the factors that facilitate coherence in the personal stories of speakers with aphasia, since aphasia does not directly affect the ability to decide which background information needs to be expressed and which shared knowledge can be left unstated.

Narrative characteristics that support the evaluative function

As noted earlier in the current review, the primary motivation for telling a story may not be to recount the narrative event per se, but rather to express the narrator's attitudes or opinions about the event and to make a point (Labov, 1972;

Polanyi, 1989). This expression of the narrator's attitudes and opinions creates interpersonal meaning (Armstrong & Ferguson, 2010). The narrator expresses his/her attitudes and opinions through narrative by (1) selecting to tell only those stories deemed to be significant or "worth telling"; and (2) highlighting or adding prominence to select information within the narrative to make one's point.

Selection of a story worth telling. One of the evaluative expectations in storytelling is that the narrated incident be "tellable" (Ochs & Capps, 2001). In other words the incident should be unusual, unexpected, unique, or remarkable (Labov & Waletzky, 1967; van Dijk, 1976). Correspondingly, personal stories will typically reflect "a struggle or polarization of some sort" (Longacre, 1996, p. 10). The very selection of which story to tell is a primary means of filling the evaluative function with one's narrative. For example, a severely apraxic member of an aphasia group once engaged the group with a humorous story about encountering a naked woman at a car wash. Such a story would not have been tellable, and thus less coherent, if the event were routine, e.g., if he had recounted that he simply went to the car wash, saw no one there, and came home.

Selection of a story worth telling is not inherently demanding on the linguistic system, so presence of aphasia does not necessarily affect one's ability to select a tellable story. In fact one of the characteristics of personal narratives of high quality is that they meet the criterion of tellability (Ulatowska, Olness, Samson, Keebler, & Goins, 2004). Tellability is consensually defined, relative to the norms of the discourse community (Bruner, 1990; van Dijk, 1976), and listeners' expectations for a tellable event increase the overall coherence of the story when the unusual elements are narrated. The evaluative content of the story can be further predicted by the ongoing topic of conversation in which it is embedded (Norrick, 2000). Personal stories that are not tellable relative to cultural expectations or the context of the conversation are often met with silence.

Clinical researchers, as well as clinicians, should use ethnographic methods to sample stories that are tellable, i.e., salient to the participants and the culture in which they interact. Otherwise it will be difficult to assess the evaluative function of personal stories in clinical settings. As a way of establishing the ecological validity of our samples, participants or clients with aphasia and their friends and family may be surveyed regarding frequency of use of personal narratives prior to stroke, favourite narrative topics, and typical audiences and co-narrators for their stories. A survey of pastimes or significant life milestones or turning points may be included, since favourite stories may be based on favourite and memorable events (Olness & Pelland, 2007). An ethnographic approach to assessing narrative functionality may also ask the narrator with aphasia and/or family to document past events or occurrences which are remembered and talked about by the participant during a given week.

Linde (1997) describes the times, places, artefacts, and regular practices that are occasions for narrative remembering, such as anniversaries, museums, photos, and holidays. Culturally shared experiences, such as the Kennedy assassination or "9/11" have also been frequently used to prompt personal narratives. One's living location and co-habitants may also predict salient narrative topics, e.g., weather stories may be common among country dwellers, and co-habitants may predict who the main characters in personal stories would be (Olness & Pelland, 2007).

Finally, certain story themes are universally salient. For example, it has been suggested that there is a set of emotions that are found in some form in every known culture: happiness, anger, sadness, fear, and disgust (Stein, Hernandez, &

Trabasso, 2008). These emotive themes may be salient prompts for personal stories. One effective way to prompt for a story is to ask, *Do you remember a time when you were [e.g., frightened/disgusted/happy]*, wait for an affirmation, then ask, *What happened?* (cf. Labov, 1972). Another way to ask is to say, *I don't know you well, but I've been told that [e.g., you had a frightening flight to Lubbock one time].* Finally, one ecological way to elicit a personal narrative is to begin by telling a brief but related narrative of one's own, e.g., *I found a mouse in my house once. Have you ever had problems with pests? Yes? What happened?*

Highlighting narrative content to make a point. The evaluative function of narrative is also filled by a process termed *narrative evaluation.* Selected information is highlighted or assigned prominence in a story to make points, and thus express the narrator's attitudes and opinions about the event. For example, in a story about a school bully the narrator may comment, *I was angry* and *The teacher's arrival was perfectly timed* as a way of implying that the narrator's anger would have resulted in a worse fate for the bully if the teacher had not arrived when she did.

Evaluative content as a whole adds to the overall coherence of personal narrative (Olness & Englebretson, 2011), and allows the narrator to express evaluative themes consistent with the topic of the narrative, such as fear, uncertainty, or restitution in a narrative of one's stroke (Armstrong & Ulatowska, 2007). One way to express evaluative content is through a separate comment apart from the event line (e.g., *I was angry* or *Her arrival was perfectly timed*). Another way is to embed evaluation within utterances (Labov, 1972) either on the event line (e.g., *This boy punched me and punched me, really HARD* or *The teacher rushed in*), or off the main event line (e.g., *I was so angry . . . I was as angry as a hornet*).

It is important to note that the number and range of evaluative devices is extensive, and drawn from multiple levels of language structure, in addition to paralinguistic devices. (See Olness et al., 2010, for a summary of several evaluative devices, as well as Labov, 1972, for the seminal work on this topic.) More important, however, is the fact that many evaluative devices are relatively non-complex linguistically, so even speakers with relatively severe aphasia have evaluative device options. Indeed, there is evidence to suggest that the types of evaluation used, their distribution in the narrative structure, and the semantic coherence of all evaluative content as a whole may be relatively preserved in narratives of speakers with aphasia, as compared to narratives of speakers without aphasia (Olness et al., 2010; Olness & Englebretson, 2011). Thus evaluation appears to be a key contributor to the overall coherence of personal stories produced by speakers with aphasia.

Some common evaluative devices that are readily used by speakers with and without aphasia include separate commentary (e.g., *This is for real!*); repetition (e.g., *Uh woman uh um rude. Rude.*); direct speech (e.g., *I go, "Say man! John sit down!"*); negation (e.g., *I couldn't use none of it*); and use of extra-high pitch on selected words (e.g., *It SEEM like it TOOK FOREVER to get that plane stopped*) (Olness et al., 2010). Note that none of these particular devices requires the use of complex language. For example, Berko-Gleason et al. (1980) comment that the relatively simple syntactic structure of direct speech may be associated with its high frequency of use by narrators with Broca's aphasia. Likewise, repetition of what one has already said or use of increased pitch does not involve any corresponding increase in linguistic complexity.

Evaluation may be found throughout the narrative superstructure, with the exception of the initiating event (Berman, 1997). For both speakers with and without aphasia, the use of evaluative devices tends to concentrate in the portions of narratives that contain the most remarkable or unusual information requiring evaluation, such as the complicating action of the story or the coda (Olness et al., 2010). For example, one narrator with moderately severe aphasia used repetition and extra modifiers to emphasise the extent of her husband's drinking problem, in the complicating action of her divorce story: *Seven days. Seven days straight* (Olness et al., 2010).

However, this ability to selectively highlight information may be diminished in relatively severe aphasia, when evaluative devices are pervasively distributed throughout the narrative (Olness et al., 2010). Evaluative devices are evaluative only when their frequency of use deviates from the baseline frequency of use (Polanyi, 1989). For example, when over-use of repetition or direct speech becomes the textual norm, these devices cease to function evaluatively. There is evidence to suggest that narratives of some speakers with more severe aphasia may overuse evaluative devices at the expense of clear referential language (Olness et al., 2010), which would in turn diminish the overall coherence of their narratives.

Coherence-building resources are interactive

The predictable narrative characteristics described above have been considered individually for their contributions to the referential and evaluative functions that together build overall narrative coherence. However, it should be emphasised that it is not the individual or additive effects of these characteristics that determine overall coherence, but rather their *combination and interaction* that builds coherent personal narratives. For example, seemingly poor personal reference in the text itself may not render a narrative incoherent if the narrator and audience share sufficient cultural background or experiences and if at least the most critical agents are clearly referenced. Likewise, even when reference is unclear, a narrator may be able to coherently evaluate his/her opinion that the event was e.g., "fearful" or "happy", which would be sufficiently coherent for a context requiring primarily evaluative coherence (e.g., an intimate interpersonal context) as opposed to a context requiring high referential coherence (e.g., a court of law). Moreover, any given form may contribute to coherence in more than one way. For example, one narrative study of reported speech, a form that can act as an evaluative device, found that many narrators with and without aphasia also used the form as an element of the main event line, and that such "dual-use" was concentrated in the complicating action (a component of narrative structure) (Ulatowska, Reyes, Santos, & Worle, 2011). Thus it is the *interaction* of coherence-building resources, and not the sum of their individual effects, that should be the primary consideration in both research and clinical accounts of the coherence of personal stories.

ASSESSING THE COHERENCE OF PERSONAL STORIES PRODUCED BY NARRATORS WITH APHASIA

We now turn to actual examples of personal narratives produced by speakers with aphasia, selected for their ability to illustrate how multi-dimensional coherence-building resources interact to support overall narrative coherence. These narratives and narrative excerpts were selected from narrative data collections of the authors, and those that can be found in publications are cited as such. Both coherent and incoherent personal stories and story excerpts told by individuals with aphasia are included, and each example is qualitatively assessed and discussed for the resource combinations that may contribute, or be lacking, towards support of overall coherence. From a clinical standpoint this would be analogous to first conducting a valid observational screening of overall discourse coherence (coherent vs incoherent), followed by identification of the potential combinations of factors that contribute to the narrative's coherence, or lack thereof, which might then lead to future "deep-testing". These examples are not intended to be comprehensive in their coverage of the full range of aphasia types, nor are they designed to represent all possible communicative contexts; descriptions of narrator characteristics and communicative contexts are detailed only to the degree that they inform the qualitative, illustrative assessment of interactions among coherence-building resources. Likewise, only those coherence-building resources that are the most relevant for each narrative example will be highlighted, rather than considering all resources for each narrative. Again, this approach is consistent with the goal of the current paper, which is to frame and illustrate issues relevant for the future development of on-line clinical analyses of narrative coherence and functionality.

Nature of the samples

Most of the following stories and story extracts were produced by middle-aged, English-speaking, Caucasian and African-American adults in the context of semi-structured interviews, following a request for a story on a topic specified by a (typically) race-matched interviewer, who in turn acted as an interested listener (Labov, 1972). Typically, the request was either to tell a personal story of a frightening experience, or to tell the story of one's stroke, often near the end of a longer discourse protocol during which interviewer and narrator had become familiar to each other. Responses were audio recorded and orthographically transcribed. Portions of the transcriptions enclosed in square brackets provide clarifications of content by the transcriptionist, or when marked "Interviewer", provide verbalisations of the Interviewer.

This approach does not necessarily account for how stories are embedded in conversation (Norrick, 2000), but it does include illustrations of how conversations are embedded in stories, in the form of direct speech (Hengst, Frame, Neuman-Stritzel, & Gannaway, 2005; Ulatowska & Olness, 2003; Ulatowska et al., 2011). The emotive and personal nature of these stories falls into the category of personally meaningful and complex functional communication that is targeted by current models of rehabilitation and rehabilitation outcomes. This sampling approach also represents those conversational contexts in which the listener cedes the floor to extend the speaker's conversational turn for the purpose of telling a personal narrative (e.g., Schegloff, 1982), including aphasia group settings in which group members take turns relating personal narratives.

Example Set 1: Multiple resources for building a coherent narrative

Multiple resources can be used by narrators with aphasia to produce coherent personal stories, even in the presence of noticeable aphasic impairment. Consider, for example, the following personal narrative of a stroke told by a middle-aged African-American man with moderate non-fluent aphasia when he was asked to relate a frightening experience (Olness & Englebretson, 2011):

> *Man it's stroke. It's comin'. Yes okay. After it's seure* [seizure]. *Uh:"!* [sound of having a seizure] *Oh Lord, oh Lord. Talking. And now, "Woo:"!* [ambulance sound] *An(d) then, "Why?" "I can't talking." It's and for, for long, not long time. Man it's angry! It angry boy. Oh. But it's okay. It's praise God.*

In a top-down fashion, the first step in assessment would be to rate the overall story as either coherent or incoherent. Despite his aphasia, this narrator's story is relatively coherent overall, i.e., the story makes sense as a whole. Next, the potential resources that contribute to coherence are considered. The topic (stroke) is clearly established at the beginning and relevant to the request for a frightening experience. With respect to the referential function, there is also a tight adherence to temporal-causal order and superstructure, which is also explicitly marked (*and now*, *and then*) and includes an evaluative coda (*But it's okay. It's praise God*). Past tense, while not explicitly marked, is assumed in narratives, so its absence does not affect coherence. Multiple factors contribute to the clear reference to agents and their activities: the small number of agents (the narrator, and perhaps the "talking" people who decided to call an ambulance); shared cultural knowledge of scripts in emergency situations (e.g., ambulances) which precludes the need for elaborate setting/background and permits use of onomatopoeia to represent the ambulance. Onomatopoeia also clarifies the poor lexical reference to the seizure. Reference to location is not stated, but is not background important to the story. Evaluation using extra comments and direct speech effectively highlights the speaker's opinions and attitude regarding stroke event and its aftermath (*Oh Lord, oh Lord*; *Why?*; *I can't talking*); repeated mention of anger; and evaluative resolution expressed in the coda *(it's okay; it's praise God*). The narrator effectively uses changes in voice pitch and quality to mark when he is using direct speech and onomatopoeia. In summary, multiple resources converge to allow both referential and evaluative functions to be filled in a coherent fashion, despite an obvious aphasic impairment.

The next passage, told by a young man with a moderate non-fluent aphasia (Ulatowska, Freedman-Stern, Doyel, Macaluso-Haynes, & North, 1983) was the passage that first prompted the second author to explore how discourse coherence can be achieved even in the presence of aphasic impairment:

> *Going to Possum Kingdom* [a regional park]. *Almost there. Other guy drunk. Head on collision. And Mike S., he was driving. And me passenger. Head on collision. And would've died. Some guy stopped along the road. And put a snorkel in my throat. And would've died. And other guy went insane. And that's it.*

Coherence is supported by a strong temporal-causal event line and superstructure, including a coda (*that's it*). The background information is relevant and shared knowledge about the park precluded the need to mention that driving was involved to get there. Shared world knowledge of road collisions, as well as unique reference to each character (*other guy, Mike S., some guy, self*), allows multiple male characters to be clearly referenced. *Snorkel* can be interpreted based on world knowledge of emergency medicine. Evaluative repetition of the comment, *would've died*, fills the evaluative function.

Sometimes lexical content can make a discourse coherent, despite impairments associated with aphasia. The following example (Freedman-Stern, Ulatowska, Baker, & DeLacoste, 1984) is an evaluative coda from a diary entry written by a man with aphasia, which illustrates this coherence-building pattern:

> *I know I was gonna be sick some day. I know it. Maybe it was for dreams I did have... Anyway I did do cripple. Yea I did sick, it was my head. Ha. I guess I had it for sixty year but I had some fun... It is to laugh. I have I am still for fun... It is to laugh. I have I am still for fun bucause* [sic] *I am still alive...*

In this passage, deficits (*sick, cripple*) are contrasted with positive aspects of life (*fun, laugh, alive*), many of which are repeated evaluatively. This coda coherently fills its evaluative function. Because the primary function of codas is to provide evaluation and close the narrative, the seemingly poor referential content has minimal negative functional impact.

Example Set 2: Poor referential function with good evaluative function

This example set provides illustrations of how, in a single narrative of a single narrator with aphasia, referential function may be poor while evaluative function may remain intact. Following is an extract of an incoherent background/setting from a personal narrative of domestic abuse told by a middle-aged Caucasian woman with moderate-severe aphasia (participant number "A-APH35" in Olness et al., 2010):

> *Tommy uh brother me. Now uh. Now uh brother, um brother uh uh side, uh side. Brother. Uh house bad. Now uh daddy um. Now. Daddy uh uh done gone. Now uh l-. Oh um. What his name? Uh Debbie. Uh uh crooked. Now. Now um uh ring, uh girl way off. No her uh seches* [: Texas]..... *Uh uh Texas. Now. Uh. Uh woma(n) uh um rude. Rude. Uh mind, uh mind lost. Uh daddy...*

Remember that a key function of the structural background/setting is referential. Despite the minimal use of verbs, progression in the event line is marked (*Now*), which supports referential coherence on the surface. However, a key contributor to referential incoherence is the poor clarity of personal reference due to sheer numbers of characters and poor verb reference to their activities, as well as the reduced morpho-syntax that restricts expression of characters' relationships.

In the excerpted closure to the same story that follows personal reference is still poor, and even though temporal reference is aided by continued adherence to temporal-causal order, the referential function is poor overall. However, the evaluative function is relatively maintained: the severity of the abuse is coherently evaluated through the use of extensive repetition, onomatopoeia, and direct speech expressing a friend's reactions, and closure with an evaluated coda (*Amen. No no. Now, uh no more*) contributes to the coherence of the evaluative content:

> *David, hurts. Hard. Blood. Everything. Uh uh look. Um, I um five. Uh uh five. And now uh blood. "What a world?"* ['What in the world happened to you?'] *Uh a friend, a friend. "Wrong?"* ["What's wrong?"] *"Porch. Uh, porch."* ["I fell off the porch."] *Angry. Mean. Now. "Oh me!" Pow! Me. Pow! Uh now blood everything. No, no! No! Uh five. Five. Uh David. Um, uh hard! Hard! Amen. No, no. Now uh no more.*

Yet another example illustrates the potential primacy of the evaluative function over the referential function in forming coherence for some speakers with aphasia. A middle-aged Caucasian man with mild aphasia told the story of his stroke twice (Olness, 2007). Tellings were separated by over a week. Excerpts from the parallel expression of the same complicating action from the two tellings are below, for comparison:

Telling 1 (Complicating action):
And, and I think that, and I went, "Goddamn it. It's something bad." I dunno. And "Damn" you know.
Telling 2 (Complicating action):
And I start, um And I start, um uh I start uh uh uh I stood up and I just, my hands hurt. And and I could read, and I could read it but I couldn't do my hand. And so I said uh "I don't wanna be like that."

Note that while both complicating actions include evaluative language such as direct speech, evaluative content completely replaces any expression of referential content in the complicating action of the first telling. Reference to agents and their activities were completely absent in the first telling of the structural complicating action, a structural location where reference to agents and their activities is most critical.

Example Set 3: Breakdown of temporal-causal order

Illustrated below is an example of a pattern found in at least two narratives of individuals with relatively more severe aphasia in the authors' data sets. Referential problems, such as anomia, hold up the progress of the event line. The narrator then cycles back to the beginning of the same portion of the event line repeated times, which disrupts the temporal-causal order. Ultimately this combination of poor reference with disruption of the temporal-causal sequencing of the narrative has a profound negative impact on the overall coherence of the narrative. In a story about an intruder, a young-elderly African-American woman with moderate anomic aphasia reiterates short portions of the event line, beginning with the direct speech of the climax. The first utterance of each iteration of the event line is underlined to display the pattern:

....And I was uh, I said, I said, "What are you doing? And when he saw I was there, when he see, when he did, when I had in there, he said. And uh, when I said something, he he said you know he said uh. I said I said, "What do you want?" That's when uh, when I was there then he, he said uh. I, I don't think he know what I wa, what you know, and what he was trying to uh, get that uh, and when I sa, when I said that and he and he saw me. And that's when he was trying to get back outside. And uh, and when, when he was trying to get the the the the, the uh [Interviewer: Door] *Door. And he was trying, he was trying, he drawin* [trying] *to he was trying to. And, and I said, "What are you doing?" That's when he come and and uh he was trying to go out then. . .* [narrative ends without resolution or coda]

ASSESSING COHERENCE OF NARRATIVES IN THEIR CONTEXT OF USE

The previous section illustrated assessment of the coherence of individual narratives elicited in clinical research settings. Considered in the current section is evaluation of narrative coherence in more naturalistic, ecologically valid contexts, which is our ultimate goal in any assessment of narrative functionality.

Assessment of narrative coherence in a group setting

Communicative competence is a primary goal of group therapy (Ewing, 2007), and expression of group members' personal experiences and opinions, e.g., through personal narratives, is a primary means of working on communicative competence in this setting (Bernstein-Ellis & Elman, 2007). Clinical researchers can document a group member's interactional achievements by examining the degree to which personal stories of a group member fit with the ongoing topic of group discussion. For example, one middle-aged African-American woman with mild aphasia (Ulatowska & Olness, 2007) made an evaluative contribution that fitted coherently with the group's joint narrative on their parallel experiences during a historic tornado:

> *Ooh, it was something to see! People running, telling, "I'm gon catch it. I'm gon catch it!" They catch that tornado, they done caught something, they catch that. They catch that tornado, they done caught something.*

Interactional achievement may be further indexed when a group member's own stories are coherent enough that subsequent stories of other group members are related to the key points made in the story he or she told.

In addition, researchers can also observe and document the interactional strategies that storytellers use to secure interest of the group; gain control of the floor; ensure understanding during their story telling; redirect and reformulate the story line or evaluative points based on interruptions, feedback, or comments from the audience; and close a story (cf. Ervin-Tripp & Küntay, 1996; Norrick, 2000). In joint story telling of co-experienced events the balance between group members' relative contributions can also be documented.

Assessment of narrative coherence in the larger cultural context

Production of coherent personal stories is dependent largely on the speaker's understanding of shared world knowledge and shared communicative resources in one's culture. As noted by Saville-Troike (2003), "while many of the functions of language are universal, the ways in which communication operates in any one society to serve these functions is language specific" (p. 14). At the discourse level, "even the definition of a well-formed discourse is determined by culture-specific rules of rhetoric" (Saville-Troike, 2003, p. 10). For example, *topic associating structure* is an alternate narrative structure sometimes used by African Americans (Michaels, 1981). As another example, a narrator's use of features of his or her native dialect can enhance the evaluative function and vividness of direct speech, as seen in the following example of an African-American woman with aphasia, who is telling the story of her stroke (Ulatowska et al., 2011):

> *I got up. I tried to get up. But I fell back down and then my daughter 'em said, "What's wrong with you Momma?" I said, "I don't know what's wrong." And they said, "Sit on down before you fall again." I said, "Shoot, it's something wrong with me." And they looked at me and said, "It sho' is."*

People can be thought of as being members of a "discourse community" (Saville-Troike, 2003, p. 17), such as members of general American culture (Polanyi, 1989) or American midwesterners (Johnstone, 1990). In research on discourse coherence and communicative competence it is essential to know the discourse community or communities (e.g., ethnic, regional, gender-based, and occupational) in which research participants are members (Saville-Troike, 2003). Likewise, it is helpful to know the cultures in which they may be participants without being a cultural member, as is the case with immigrants. Such information provides one window into the pre-morbid discourse practices of our clinical research participants and the communicative demands placed on them, against which we can assess their post-stroke performance. For example, for one man with aphasia whose Bantu culture places value on intergenerational transmission of one's values through stories, narratives were one means by which he transmitted his cultural heritage to his grandchildren (Ulatowska & Self, 1996).

The "culture of assessment" should be equally considered as a discourse culture, for the discourse-testing contexts may be alien to our research participants and clients. For example, in research by the second author, evidence of this cultural disparity was seen in post-testing reactions of American participants to some picture-elicited discourse tasks, and differential willingness of Europeans and Americans to share personal narratives with a relative stranger. We have attempted to bridge this cultural disparity gap by including interviewers who are from the same cultural group as the client with aphasia, and through sampling of discourse on universally salient themes, such as a frightening experience or the story of one's stroke.

Notably, only a certain percentage of members of a discourse culture are considered "good storytellers" by members of that culture (Olness, Ulatowska, Carpenter, Williams-Hubbard & Dykes, 2005; Ulatowska, Olness, Samson, et al., 2004). Thus clinical research design should include ethnographic descriptions of participants' pre-morbid storytelling abilities and practices within their respective cultures. Notably, the general characteristics of stories culturally rated as "good" include selection of more salient topics, conventional narrative structure, and use of drama-like features such as direct speech, prosodic shifts, voice changes, and repetition. Many of these storytelling features are preserved in narrators with aphasia (Olness et al., 2010), so aphasic narrators who were good storytellers before their strokes may be able to build on their pre-morbid storytelling abilities.

CONCLUSIONS AND CODA

Longacre (1996) comments that it is preferable to study discourse "in action as a functioning organism" (p. 31). The qualitative framework and illustrative assessments of personal stories provided by the current review were motivated by a desire to explore how linguistic forms, narrative structures, shared knowledge, and communicative context *function together* in the production of coherent stories, as a complement to the many quantitative discourse studies of forms and structures that the field of discourse aphasiology has mastered and whose ecological significance we are working to understand (Armstrong, 2000). As noted by Damico, Simmons-Mackie, and Schweitzer (1995), "qualitative research offers an alternative approach for specific questions that is as valid and valuable as more quantitative and experimentally oriented research" (p. 90). Our hope is that the current review lives up to this potential, and that the issues that this review raises may guide the field towards selection of complementary quantitative approaches that hold the most promise for elucidating narrative functionality. A logical next step in development of on-line transcription-less approaches to analysis would be to assess the reliability and external validity of behavioural observations and qualitative ratings. For instance, the field may choose to check the reliability of qualitative transcription-free ratings of referential functions and to test their convergent validity with transcription-bound analyses of cohesion. Similarly, on-line ratings of overall evaluative functionality and point making may be validated with transcription-dependent analysis of evaluative device use. Quantitative measures, carefully chosen to focus on those resources and resource combinations that play a key role in the building of overall narrative coherence and functionality, may provide the "deep test" that helps establish the validity of more clinically feasible transcription-less approaches.

For speakers with aphasia there is high potential for communicative competence in storytelling and the many intrapersonal and interpersonal functions it fills, yet aphasia also poses a threat to this competence. When someone with aphasia is unable to "tell their own story" they need the opportunity to have intrapersonal and interpersonal needs met through joint telling of stories, and through listening to personal stories of others. However, if researchers and clinicians in our field can find a way to guide narrators with aphasia in fulfilling their own autobiographical need for expression, we can hope to have made at least a small contribution to their lives.

Certainly people who have aphasia will define for us those storytelling contexts which are the most meaningful for them, and those where they have their greatest struggles. What may be "incoherent" to researchers in a clinical context may very well be fully coherent and meaningful in the contexts of aphasic persons' lives. The goal in many interpersonal communication contexts may not be full referential clarity, but rather effective expression of one's opinion, as expressed through evaluation. As Norrick (2000) notes, tellers of personal stories "re-create memories of past events to fit the present context" (p. 2), but defining the most functional of storytelling contexts will require consultation with the real experts. Audrey Holland (2010) writes about her lifelong process of learning about aphasia from the experts who live with the disorder. As one local friend and clinician, who has spent her whole life working with this population, recently commented, "I have learned more about aphasia from being friends with these folks than I ever began to know . . . the disorder is more pervasive, changes lives more dramatically, than I imagined. Living with aphasia (or in my case, hanging out with aphasic persons) . . . is the way to really learn about it."

REFERENCES

AphasiaBank. (2011). Retrieved from http://www.talkbank.org/AphasiaBank/ (accessed 14 January 2011).

Aphasia Corner Blog. (2011). Retrieved from http://aphasiacorner.com/blog/ (accessed 14 January 2011).

Armstrong, E. (1997). *A grammatical analysis of aphasic discourse: Changes in meaning-making over time* (PhD thesis). Macquarie University, Sydney, Australia.

Armstrong, E. (2000). Aphasic discourse analysis: The story so far. *Aphasiology*, *9*, 872–892.

Armstrong, E., & Ferguson, A. (2010). Language, meaning, context, and functional communication. *Aphasiology*, *24*, 480–496.

Armstrong, E., & Ulatowska, H. K., (2007). Stroke stories: Conveying emotive experiences in aphasia. In M. J. Ball & J. S. Damico (Eds.), *Clinical aphasiology: Future directions*. New York, NY: Psychology Press.

Armstrong, L., Brady, M., Mackenzie, C., & Norrie, J. (2007). Transcription-less analysis of aphasic discourse: A clinician's dream or a possibility? *Aphasiology*, *21*, 355–374.

Bastiaanse, R., & Zonneveld, R. (1998). On the relation between verb inflection and verb position in Dutch agrammatic aphasics. *Brain and Language*, *64*, 165–181.

Berko-Gleason, J., Goodglass, H., Obler, L., Green, E., Hyde, M. R., & Weintraub, B. (1980). Narrative strategies of aphasic and normal-speaking subjects. *Journal of Speech and Hearing Resesarch*, *30*, 370–382.

Berman, R. A. (1997). Narrative theory and narrative development: The Labovian impact. *Journal of Narrative and Life History*, *7*, 235–244.

Bernstein-Ellis, E., & Elman, R. J. (2007). Aphasia group treatment: The aphasia center of California approach. In R. J. Elman (Ed.), *Group treatment of neurogenic communication disorders: The expert clinician's approach, 2nd edition* (pp. 71–94). San Diego, CA: Plural Publishing.

Bruner, J. (1990). *Acts of meaning*. Cambridge, MA: Harvard University Press.

Cherney, L. R., Halper, A. S., Holland, A. L., & Cole, R (2008). Computerized script training for aphasia: Preliminary results. *American Journal of Speech-Language Pathology*, *17*, 19–34.

Cherney, L. R., Shadden, B. B., & Coelho, C. A. (1998). *Analyzing discourse in communicatively impaired adults*. Gaithersburg, MD: Aspen Publishers.

Christiansen, J. A. (1995). Coherence violations and propositional usage in the narratives of fluent aphasics. *Brain and Language, 51*, 291–317.

Damico, J. S., Simmons-Mackie, N. N., & Schweitzer, L. A. (1995). Addressing the third law of gardening: Methodological alternative in aphasiology. In M. L. Lemme (Ed.), *Clinical aphasiology, Volume 23* (pp. 83–93). Austin, TX: Pro-Ed.

Dollaghan, C. A. (2007). *The handbook for evidence-based practice in communication disorders*. Baltimore, MD: Paul H. Brooks Publishing.

Edwards, S., & Bastiaanse, R. (1998). Diversity in the lexical and syntactic abilities of fluent aphasic speakers. *Aphasiology, 12*, 99–117.

Elman, R. J., & Bernstein-Ellis, E. (1995). What is functional? *American Journal of Speech-Language Pathology, 4*, 115–117.

Ervin-Tripp, S., & Küntay, A. (1996). The occasioning and structure of conversational stories. In T. Givón (Ed.), *Conversation: Cognitive, communicative and social perspectives* (pp. 133–166). Amsterdam, The Netherlands: John Benjamins.

Ewing, S. E. A. (2007). Group process, group dynamics, and group techniques with neurogenic communication disorders. In R. J. Elman (Ed.), *Group treatment of neurogenic communication disorders: The expert clinician's approach, 2nd edition* (pp. 11–23). San Diego, CA: Plural Publishing.

Frank. A. W. (1997). *The wounded storyteller: Body, illness, and ethics*. Chicago, IL: University of Chicago Press.

Freedman-Stern, R., Ulatowska, H. K., Baker, T., & DeLacoste, C. (1984). Disruption of written language in aphasia: A case study. *Brain and Language, 22*, 181–205.

Garrett, K. L., & Pimentel, J. T. (2007). Measuring outcomes of group therapy. In R. J. Elman (Ed.), *Group treatment of neurogenic communication disorders: The expert clinician's approach, 2nd edition* (pp. 25–61). San Diego, CA: Plural Publishing.

Glosser, G. (1993). Discourse production patterns in neurologically impaired and aged populations. In H. H. Brownell & Y. Joanette (Eds.), *Narrative discourse in neurologically impaired and normal aging adults* (pp. 191–211). San Diego, CA: Singular Publishing Group.

Glosser, G., & Deser, T. (1990). Patterns of discourse production among neurological patients with fluent language disorders. *Brain and Language, 40*, 67–88.

Halliday, M. A. K., & Hasan, R. (1976). *Cohesion in English*. London, UK: Longman.

Hengst, J. A., Frame, S. R., Neuman-Stritzel, T., & Gannaway, R. (2005). Using others' words: Conversational use of reported speech by individuals with aphasia and their communication partners. *Journal of Speech, Language and Hearing Research, 48*, 137–156.

Holland, A. (1977). Some practical considerations in aphasia rehabilitation. In M. Sullivan & M. S. Kommers (Eds.), *Rationale for adult aphasia therapy* (pp. 167–180). Lincoln, NE: University of Nebraska Medical Center Print Shop.

Holland, A. L. (2007). The power of aphasias groups: Celebrating Roger Ross. In R. J. Elman (Ed.), *Group treatment of neurogenic communication disorders: The expert clinician's approach, 2nd edition* (pp. 249–253). San Diego, CA: Plural Publishing.

Holland, A. (2010). Lessons from a clinical life in aphasia. *Topics in Stroke Rehabilitation, 17*, 13–19.

Huber, W. (1990). Text comprehension and production in aphasia: Analysis in terms of micro- and macrostructure. In Y. Joanette & H. Brownell (Eds.), *Discourse ability and brain damage: Theoretical and empirical perspectives* (pp. 154–179). New York, NY: Springer-Verlag.

Jakobson, R. (1990). *On language* (L. R. Waugh & M. Monville-Burston, Eds.). Cambridge, MA: Harvard University Press.

Johnstone, B. (1990). *Stories, community, and place: Narratives from middle America*. Bloomington: Indiana University Press.

Kenyon, G. M. (2006). Biography. In *The encyclopedia of aging, 4th edition, Volume 1, A–K* (pp. 112–114). New York, NY: Springer Publishing.

Kleinman, A. (1988). *The illness narratives: Suffering, healing, and the human condition*. New York, NY: Basic Books.

Labov, W. (1972). *Language in the inner city: Studies in the black English vernacular*. Philadelphia: University of Pennsylvania Press.

Labov, W. (1997). Some further steps in narrative analysis. *Journal of Narrative and Life History, 7*, 395–415.

Labov, W., & Waletzky, J. (1967). Narrative analysis: Oral versions of personal experience. In J. Helm (Ed.), *Essays of the verbal and visual arts: Proceedings of the 1966 annual spring meeting of the American Ethnological Society* (pp. 12–44). Seattle: University of Washington Press.

Linde, C. (1997). Narrative: Experience, memory, folklore. *Journal of Narrative and Life History*, *7*, 281–289.

Longacre, R. E. (1996). *The grammar of discourse, 2nd edition.* New York, NY: Plenum Press.

Mandler, J. M. (1984). *Stories, scripts and scenes: Aspects of schema theory.* Hillsdale, NJ: Lawrence Erlbaum Associates.

Michaels, S. (1981). "Sharing time": Children's narrative styles and differential access to literacy. *Language in Society*, *10*(3), 423–442.

Norrick, N. R. (2000). *Conversational narrative: Storytelling in everyday talk.* Amsterdam, The Netherlands: John Benjamins Publishing.

Ochs, E., & Capps, L. (2001). *Living narrative: Creating lives in everyday storytelling.* Cambridge, MA: Harvard University Press.

Olness, G. S. (2006). Genre, verb, and coherence in picture-elicited discourse of adults with aphasia. *Aphasiology*, *20*, 175–187.

Olness, G. S. (2007, May). *Narrative structure in aphasia: Impact of task and aphasia severity.* Platform presentation at the 2007 Clinical Aphasiology Conference, Scottsdale, Arizona.

Olness, G. S., & Englebretson, E. F. (2011). On the coherence of information highlighted by narrators with aphasia. *Aphasiology*, *25*(6–7), 713–726.

Olness, G. S., Matteson, S. E., & Stewart, C. T. (2010). "Let me tell you the point": How speakers with aphasia assign prominence to information in narratives. *Aphasiology*, *24*, 697–708.

Olness, G. S., & Pelland, D. L. (2007, February). *Narrative topic and evaluation as expressions of ethnicity and self-identity in aphasia.* Poster presented at the 2007 Texas Research Symposium on Language Diversity, Austin, Texas.

Olness, G. S., Ulatowska, H. K., Carpenter, C. M., Williams-Hubbard, L. J., & Dykes, J. C. (2005). Holistic assessment of narrative quality: A social validation study. *Aphasiology*, *29*, 251–262.

Polanyi, L. (1989). *Telling the American story: A structural and cultural analysis of conversational storytelling.* Cambridge, MA: MIT.

Randall, W. L., & Kenyon, G. M. (2001). *Ordinary wisdom: Biographical aging and the journey of life.* Westport, CT: Pareger.

Sacks, O. (2010). *The mind's eye. Chapter 2: Recalled to life* (pp. 32–52). New York, NY: Alfred A. Knopf.

Saville-Troike, M. (2003). *The ethnography of communication: An introduction.* Malden, MA: Blackwell Publishing.

Schegloff, E. A. (1982). Discourse as interactional achievement: Some uses of "uh huh" and other things that come between sentences. In D. Tannen (Ed.), *Georgetown University Round Table on Languages and Linguistics. Analyzing discourse: Text and talk* (pp. 71–93). Washington, DC: Georgetown University Press.

Shadden, B. (2005). Aphasia as identity theft: Theory and practice. *Aphasiology*, *19*, 211–223.

Schank, R. C., & Abelson, R. P. (1977). *Scripts, plans, goals, and understanding.* Hillsdale, NJ: Lawrence Erlbaum Associates.

Stein, N. L., Hernandez, M. W., & Trabasso, T. (2008). Advances in modeling emotion and thought: The importance of developmental, online, and multilevel analyses. In M. Lewis, J. M. Haviland-Jones, & L. F. Barrett (Eds.) *Handbook of emotions* (3rd ed., pp. 574–586). New York, NY: The Guilford Press.

StoryCorps. (2010). www.storycorps.org (accessed 14 January 2011).

Ulatowska, H. K. (2010). Journey through narratives: The unexpected vistas. In B. Bokus (Ed.), *Studies in the psychology of language and communication* (pp. 135–147). Warsaw, Poland: Matrix Publishers.

Ulatowska, H. K., Allard, L., & Chapman, S. B. (1990). Narrative and procedural discourse in aphasia. In Y. Joanette & H. H. Brownell (Eds.), *Discourse ability and brain damage: Theoretical and empirical perspectives* (pp. 180–198). New York, NY: Springer-Verlag.

Ulatowska, H. K., Freedman-Stern, R., Doyel, A. W., Macaluso-Haynes, S., & North, A. J. (1983). Production of narrative discourse in aphasia. *Brain and Language*, *19*, 317–334.

Ulatowska, H. K., & Olness, G. S. (2001) Dialectal variants of verbs in narratives of African Americans with aphasia: Some methodological considerations. In M. Paradis (Ed.), *Manifestations of aphasia symptoms in different languages* (pp. 9–26). Amsterdam, The Netherlands: Pergamon.

Ulatowska, H. K., & Olness, G. S. (2003). On the nature of direct speech in narratives of African Americans with aphasia. *Brain and Language*, *87*, 69–70.

Ulatowska, H. K. & Olness, G. S. (2004). Discourse. *The MIT encyclopedia of communication disorders* (pp. 300–302). Cambridge, MA: The MIT Press.

Ulatowska, H. K., & Olness, G. S. (2007). Pragmatics in discourse performance: Insights from aphasiology. *Seminars in Speech-Language Pathology*, *28*, 148–157.

Ulatowska, H. K., Olness, G. S., Samson, A. M., Keebler, M. W, & Goins, K. E. (2004). On the nature of personal narratives of high quality. *Advances in Speech-Language Pathology*, *6*, 3–14.

Ulatowska, H. K., Olness, G. S., Wertz, R. T., & Hill, C. L. (2002). Patterns of verb use in narratives of African Americans with aphasia. *Brain and Language*, *83*, 57–59.

Ulatowska, H. K., Olness, G. S., & Williams, L. J. (2004). Coherence of narratives in aphasia. *Brain and Language*, *71*, 249–251.

Ulatowska, H. K., Reyes, B. A., Santos, T. O., & Worle, C. (2011). Stroke narratives in aphasia: The role of reported speech. *Aphasiology*, *25*, 93–105.

Ulatowska, H. K., & Self, S. T. (1996). Is ethnographic assessment a reality in aphasia? *Aphasiology*, *10*, 494–496.

Van Dijk, T. A. (1976). Philosophy of action and theory of narrative. *Poetics*, *5*, 287–338.

Van Dijk, T. A., & Kintsch, W. (1983). *Strategies of discourse comprehension*. New York, NY: Academic Press.

APHASIOLOGY, 2011, 25 (11), 1414–1430

Lexical diversity for adults with and without aphasia across discourse elicitation tasks

Gerasimos Fergadiotis and Heather Harris Wright

Department of Speech and Hearing Science, Arizona State University, Tempe, AZ, USA

Background: Differences in lexical diversity (LD) across different discourse elicitation tasks have been found in neurologically intact adults (NIA) (Fergadiotis, Wright, & Capilouto, 2010) but have not been investigated systematically in people with aphasia (PWA). Measuring lexical diversity in PWA may serve as a useful clinical tool for evaluating the impact of word retrieval difficulties at the discourse level.
Aims: The study aims were (a) to explore the differences between the oral language samples of PWA and NIA in terms of LD as measured by dedicated computer software (*voc-D*), (b) to determine whether PWA are sensitive to discourse elicitation task in terms of LD, and (c) to identify whether differences between PWA and NIA vary in magnitude as a function of discourse task.
Method & Procedures: Oral language samples from 25 PWA and 27 NIA were analysed. Participants completed three commonly used discourse elicitation tasks (single pictures, sequential pictures, story telling) and voc-*D* was used to obtain estimates of their LD.
Outcomes & Results: A mixed 2 × 3 ANOVA revealed a significant group × task interaction that was followed by an investigation of simple main effects and tetrad comparisons. Different patterns of LD were uncovered for each group. For the NIA group results were consistent with previous findings in the literature according to which LD varies as a function of elicitation technique. However, for PWA sequential pictures and story telling elicited comparable estimates of LD.
Conclusions: Results indicated that LD is one of the microlinguistic indices that are influenced by elicitation task and the presence of aphasia. These findings have important implications for modelling lexical diversity and selecting and interpreting results from different discourse elicitation tasks.

Keywords: Discourse; Productive vocabulary; Computational linguistics.

An important aspect of aphasia assessment is the analysis of discourse production. Discourse is successfully produced when the listener is able to reconstruct the message sent and interpret its intended meaning. People with aphasia (PWA) present with word retrieval deficits that can significantly impact how successfully their discourse

Address correspondence to: Heather Harris Wright, Arizona State University, Department of Speech and Hearing Science, P.O. Box 870102, Tempe, AZ 85287-0102, USA. E-mail: heather.wright.1@asu.edu

This research was partially supported by the National Institute on Aging Grant R01AG029476. We are especially grateful to the study participants. We also thank the volunteers in the Aging and Adult Language Lab at ASU for assistance with transcription and language analyses, and Leonid Spector, Davida Fromm, and Margaret Forbes from Carnegie Mellon University for assisting with CLAN coding and facilitating exchange of data.

http://dx.doi.org/10.1080/02687038.2011.603898

production is conveyed. For example, their verbal output may include non-referential terms, fillers, paraphasias, and/or neologisms. Discourse analysis offers an opportunity to observe and study, through a wide variety of analyses, these complex cognitive/linguistic behaviours in the most naturally occurring and commonly used form of communication. As such, language sample analysis has been used as a clinical tool for differential diagnosis (e.g., Fleming & Harris, 2008; Murray, 2009), a key indicator for determining the efficacy of treatment approaches for individuals with aphasia (e.g., Cameron, Wambaugh, Wright, & Nessler, 2006; del Toro et al., 2008; Rider, Wright, Marshall, & Page, 2008); as well as an indicator of social validity (e.g., Ballard & Thompson, 1999).

Microlinguistic processes that give rise to specific discourse features, such as lexical-semantics, can be evaluated with different content analyses. These techniques may include assessments of informativeness, efficiency, and lexical diversity (LD) of a speaker's production. Reduced informativeness and reduced efficiency have been well documented in the aphasia literature with different discourse elicitation techniques. In addition, these properties have been explored in PWA speaking different languages, ranging in severity of language impairment, and ranging in time post onset of aphasia (Honda, Mitachi, & Wafamori, 1999; Larfeuil & Dorze, 1997; McNeil, Doyle, Fossett, Park, & Goda, 2001; McNeil et al., 2007). LD has also been quantified in PWA but less frequently and often estimated incorrectly.

LEXICAL DIVERSITY IN DISCOURSE PRODUCTION BY PWA

For the purposes of this study, LD will be defined within Chapelle's (1994) model of vocabulary. Chapelle's model consists of four dimensions: (a) vocabulary size, (b) word knowledge (e.g., phonology, syntactic properties, etc), (c) density of the semantic network, and (d) processes that are involved in lexical access and retrieval. Within this framework, language performance is assumed to depend on both the implicit knowledge one possesses (e.g., variety of vocabulary) and the mechanisms that allow her/him to process it (e.g., access and retrieval). What becomes evident, then, is that *knowledge of* vocabulary and the *capacity to* demonstrate that knowledge cannot be equated (Chomsky, 1980). Based on these premises LD can be defined as the range of vocabulary deployed in a text by a speaker that reflects his/her capacity to access and retrieve target words from a relatively intact knowledge base (i.e., lexicon) for the construction of higher linguistic units. It is noteworthy that this view of LD is consistent with "performance" definitions that de-emphasise loss of language knowledge as the primary deficit in aphasia which is instead recast as an access deficit (e.g., McNeil & Pratt, 2001).

The efficiency of lexical access during discourse production depends on the synergy of several highly dynamical systems (Bock, 1982; Dell, 1986; Levelt, 1989) that may be impaired in PWA. Word retrieval depends on lexical characteristics (e.g., word frequency) and the interaction at different linguistic levels (e.g., phonologic, semantic, syntactic) of competing items in the lexicon. For example, Gordon and Dell (2003) have suggested that at the lemma selection stage of sentence generation (Levelt, Roelofs, & Meyer, 1999) at which words are selected as semantic/syntactic entities (Kempen & Hoenkamp, 1987), the selection of competing lexical targets depends on two separate networks. First, as the sentence unfolds, semantic nodes set off a target along with multiple semantic competitors through spreading activation. Subsequently, lexical items receive input from a network that applies syntactic constraints. During the same stage, phonologically related competitors may interfere further with the selection of target words (Schwartz, Dell, Martin, Gahl, & Sobel, 2006 in Dell, Oppenheim, & Kilttredge, 2008). In addition, the selection of the appropriate vocabulary may be influenced by supralinguistic factors such as the topic of the discourse, the genre a speaker chooses to respond, and the interlocutors (Haliday & Hassan, 1989). The relative strength of the signal that comes from different sources eventually determines the selection of linguistic representations.

Disruptions in one or more of these mechanisms can have direct effects on word retrieval during discourse production. Omissions can occur after a failure of the system to make words reach their activation threshold. Or paraphasias may be observed when competitors prevail over the target words. This interference from competition may arise from different sources. So, in "The cat eats the cheese", the selection of "cat" might be hindered from semantic or phonological competitors such as "dog" or "rat". Or interference may arise from other words in the sentence or the broader context in which the phrase occurs. Also, according to Gordon and Dell's *division of labour hypothesis* (2003), a lesion in the network responsible for boosting or inhibiting syntactic representations (or in the semantic network) can influence the ease with which certain lexical items are retrieved. Although it may often be difficult to pinpoint the exact mechanism of lexical processing breakdown, the nature and extent of impairment can potentially influence the range of vocabulary a speaker exhibits.

MEASURING LEXICAL DIVERSITY

The most obvious way to capture LD in a sample would be to count the number of different words (NDW or *types*). However, only when the number of total words (*tokens*) is kept constant, are comparisons of NDW across different samples meaningful. Otherwise the NDW would reflect both LD as well as the contribution of length; that is, individuals who produced more verbal output would be credited with higher LD. To overcome this obstacle one could consider the ratio of the types divided by the tokens (TTR) to control for length. However, even though TTR is an improvement compared to the NDW, it is still inherently flawed because it also varies as a function of sample length. As the sample increases the probability of introducing new words decreases; and as a result the growth of the numerator in the TTR decelerates. However, the denominator (i.e., the number of tokens) always increases steadily with every additional word and as a result, overall, the TTR decreases monotonically. Therefore comparisons across speakers or even across different samples produced by the same speaker will be confounded by sample length. In an example that highlights the central weakness of TTR, McNeil et al. (2007) found that their participants with aphasia had significantly lower TTR on the Story Retelling Procedure (SRP; Doyle et al., 1998) compared to other discourse samples (e.g., procedural descriptions). McNeil et al. acknowledged that sample length variations might have contributed to this counterintuitive finding. Indeed, given that the number of words elicited using the SRP was significantly greater than any other elicitation procedure, lower TTR were expected.

To solve similar problems, researchers have used various algebraic transformations of TTR—e.g., Split TTR (Engber, 1995); Root TTR (Guiraud, 1960), Corrected TTR (Carroll, 1964), Log TTR (Herdan, 1960)—some of which have been applied to language samples produced by adults with aphasia (e.g., Prins, Snow, & Wagenaar, 1978; Wachal & Spreen, 1973). In these studies PWA produced significantly less lexically diverse samples compared to their NI counterparts. However, some of these tools have also been found to covary with sample length, thus yielding mathematically and conceptually spurious results. Others require very large samples to produce stable estimates that prohibit their use with PWA (Jarvis, 2002; Malvern & Richards, 1997; Tweedie & Baayen, 1998; Vermeer, 2000).

To overcome these difficulties, some researchers have proposed standardising sample size through truncation. However, even though "standard" lengths have been proposed (Brookshire & Nicholas, 1994; Prins & Bastiaanse, 2004) often it is not feasible to obtain a predetermined number of tokens across studies. One reason is that sample length may depend on the elicitation task. When individuals describe a single picture or a procedure such as planting a flower in the garden, NIA and PWA often produce samples that are less than 200 tokens (Nicholas & Brookshire, 1993; Wright & Capilouto, 2011). It is common, then, for researchers to ignore consensus and restrict the number of tokens to be equal to the shortest sample in the study. As an example, Gordon (2008) used samples that consisted of 200 content word tokens. An additional issue that arises with truncation is that discarding any amount of a language sample reduces the samples' integrity and therefore reduces the validity of the analysis (McCarthy & Jarvis, 2010). Rather, it is possible that restricting the sample might obscure the findings due to clustering of content words (Prins & Bastiaanse, 2004).

Recently a new measure, *D*, was developed that combines an algebraic transformation model and curve fitting to estimate LD. *D* appears to be relatively robust to length variation, a feature that allows for comparisons of discourse samples within and between participants as well as across studies (McKee, Malvern, & Richards, 2000) without requiring truncation. The validity of *D* has been explored in several studies and has been found to be satisfactory (Malvern & Richards, 1997; McCarthy & Jarvis, 2010; McKee et al., 2000). *D* can be estimated using the voc-*D* program in Computerised Language Analysis (CLAN; MacWhinney, 2000) and the process is reasonably automated and straightforward once the samples have been transcribed.

EFFECTS OF LANGUAGE SAMPLING TECHNIQUE

A variety of elicitation techniques have been used to obtain language samples. For example, researchers have asked participants to describe single or sequential pictorial stimuli (Christiansen, 1995; Nicholas & Brookshire 1993; Olness, 2006; Wright & Capilouto, 2009). Further, narratives have been elicited through re-telling of familiar stories (i.e., story tellings) and/or sharing past experiences through personal narratives (Ash et al., 2006; Coelho, Grela, Corso, Gamble, & Feinn, 2005; Hough & Barrow, 2003; Ulatowska, North, & Macaluso-Haynes, 1981). It is generally accepted that different elicitation techniques may impose different cognitive and linguistic demands (Bliss & McCabe, 2006; Brady, Armstrong, & Mackenzie, 2005; Nicholas & Brookshire, 1993; Ulatowska, Allard, & Chapman, 1990). For example, tasks may facilitate lexical access if they are associated with a high propensity for eliciting concrete, high-imageability, and high-frequency words or if they provide rich contextual information (Balota & Chumbley, 1984; Grosjean, 1980; Kroll & Merves, 1986; Tyler & Wessels, 1983). As a result, the performance on some microlinguistic indices such as LD may vary depending on the discourse type or the elicitation technique.

In a recent study Fergadiotis et al. (2010) investigated the effect of various elicitation techniques, and the discourse type most often elicited by them, on LD in cognitively healthy adults. Four discourse tasks were included; procedures, eventcasts, story telling, and recounts. Procedures are activity-focused, step-by-step descriptions of how to achieve a goal (e.g., how to plant a flower; Longacre, 1996). The other three tasks were designed to elicit three different types of narrative discourse. Eventcasts are narratives that explain a scene of activities (e.g., Cookie Theft Picture), stories are fictionaliSed, highly structured forms (e.g., Cinderella), and recounts are verbal reiterations of an event (e.g., what one did last weekend) (Heath, 1986). Study participants included 86 cognitively healthy adults comprising two age groups: young (20–29 years old) and old (70–89 years old). Using *D* as the method for estimating LD, Fergadiotis et al. found a LD hierarchy that was similar across age groups for the four discourse types. Procedural discourse yielded the lowest LD followed by eventcasts and story telling, with recounts yielding the highest *D* values. Fergadiotis et al. concluded that, in cognitively healthy adults, LD varies as a function of elicitation technique and discourse type.

Wright, Silverman, and Newhoff (2003) measured TTR, NDW, and *D* in picture descriptions produced by adults with fluent and nonfluent aphasia. Sample length, measured by number of words, varied across the two aphasia groups. When sample length was not controlled, the participants with fluent aphasia yielded significantly higher *D* and NDW values compared to the participants with nonfluent aphasia indicating greater LD in their discourse samples. Once samples were truncated to 100 and 200 word samples, groups differed significantly for all measures (i.e., TTR, NDW, *D*). According to Wright et al., the findings demonstrate that *D* is a sensitive measure of subtle differences in LD in adults with aphasia that are not detected by TTR. Further, *D* is not as sensitive to input sample size as TTR is. However, the study included only one discourse elicitation task and a small number of study participants ($N = 9$ per group).

The current study aims to expand on Fergadiotis et al.'s and Wright et al.'s work by: (a) establishing whether there are differences between the oral language samples of PWA and NIA in terms of LD as measured by a novel approach, (b) determining whether PWA are sensitive to discourse elicitation task in terms of LD, and (c) identifying whether differences between PWA and NIA vary in magnitude as a function of discourse task. Based on the well-documented word retrieval difficulties experienced by PWA that can severely affect their discourse production it is anticipated that language samples of PWA will demonstrate lower LD across all discourse tasks compared to NIA. Further, based on the effect of discourse task on LD in NIA, it is hypothesised that PWA will also demonstrate differences across tasks. Finally, we predict that when language samples are elicited using story telling, PWA will demonstrate poorer LD in the samples compared to the NIA group due to the increased demands that are associated with this elicitation technique.

METHOD

Participants

Language samples from 27 PWA with mild to moderate level of aphasia severity were retrieved from AphasiaBank, an online shared database that collects and analyses digital recordings of discourse from PWA across a series of tasks. All participants had acquired aphasia secondary to a single left hemisphere stroke. In addition, PWA met criteria for the study that included (a) chronic aphasia (minimum = 11 months post onset of stroke and maximum = 164 months), (b) no reported history of psychiatric or neurodegenerative disorders, (c) aided or unaided normal hearing acuity, (d) corrected or uncorrected normal visual acuity, (e) English as their primary language, and

(f) classification of anomic or conduction aphasia as determined by performance on the *Western Aphasia Battery-Revised* (*WAB-R*; Kertesz, 2007). Further, several subtests from the *Reading Comprehension Battery for Aphasia, Second Edition* (*RCBA–2*; LaPointe & Horner, 1998) were administered as part of the AphasiaBank protocol but these were not analysed for the current study.

Only individuals with either anomic or conduction aphasia from AphasiaBank were included for several reasons. First, we were interested in obtaining a relatively large, yet homogeneous sample that would allow us to study LD in relative isolation from other impaired production processes. For example, individuals with nonfluent aphasias often exhibit deficits of articulatory-phonetic nature that render the coding of paraphasias difficult (e.g., apraxia of speech; Dell, Schwartz, Martin, Saffran, & Gagnon, 1997; McNeil, 1997). Second, estimating LD using voc-*D* requires a minimum of 50 tokens and therefore the inclusion of individuals with nonfluent aphasia who sometimes demonstrate very limited verbal output could become problematic.

All language samples for the NIA group came from an ongoing study of normal discourse under the direction of one of the authors (HHW). These participants were selected to closely match the PWA in terms of gender, age, and years of education. In addition they met the following inclusion criteria for participation in the study: (a) no history of stroke, head injury, or neurogenic disorder, per self-report, (b) aided or unaided hearing acuity within normal limits; (c) normal or corrected visual acuity; (d) monolingual speakers of English; (e) normal cognitive functioning as indicated by performance on the *Mini Mental State Examination* (*MMSE*; Folstein, Folstein, & McHugh, 1975); and (f) no signs of depression as indicated by a passing score (0–4) on the *Geriatric Depression Scale* (Brink et al., 1982). All participants lived independently and were recruited from the Lexington, KY and Phoenix, AZ communities. Table 1 summarises participants' characteristics.

Discourse elicitation

Stimuli and instructions. Discourse samples were collected in a single session and three commonly used tasks for eliciting discourse for clinical and research purposes were employed: sequential pictures, single pictures, and telling of the story of *Cinderella* (Grimes, 2005). The three tasks were designed to elicit two different types of

TABLE 1
Participant characteristics

	PWA group (*N = 27*)	*NIA group* (*N = 27*)
Age (yrs)	*M* = 66.81 (*SD* = *12.83*)	*M* = 67.45 (*SD* = *13.20*)
Gender	19 males, 8 females	19 males, 8 females
Education	*M* = 15.72 (*SD* = *3.72*)	*M* = 15.02 (*SD* = *3.56*)
WAB-R[1] Aphasia type	Anomic = 19	
Type	Conduction = 8	
WAB-R AQ[2]	*M* = 76.82 (*SD* = *9.83*)	
BNT[3]	*M* = 7.45 (*SD* = *4.25*)	

[1]Western Aphasia Battery – Revised;
[2]Western Aphasia Battery – Revised Aphasia Quotient;
[3]Boston Naming Test.

narrative discourse: eventcasts using the former two and story telling using the latter. The sequential picture stimuli included a four-frame strip from Menn et al. (1998) and a six-frame cartoon strip. The first is referred to as "*Broken Window*" and depicts a boy kicking a ball; the ball goes through a closed window and knocks down a lamp before a man picks up the ball and looks out of the window. The second, referred to as "*Umbrella*" depicts the story of a student who refuses to take the umbrella his mother offers him as he leaves for school; on his way to school it starts raining and he returns home to take the umbrella.

The single picture stimuli each showed a situation with a central theme and animate and inanimate pictured elements interacting. Each picture implied temporal sequencing of events prior and after the pictured scene. One of the single pictures is a photograph by Annie Wells of an emergency rescue of a girl from flood waters (Rubin & Newton, 2001). The second single picture stimulus is Nicholas and Brookshire's "*Cat Rescue*" (Nicholas & Brookshire, 1993). In this picture a little girl's cat is in a tree and her dad has tried to rescue the cat but got stuck in the tree; the fire department is arriving to rescue the cat and the man from the tree. The single and sequential picture stimuli can be found at: www.talkbank.org/AphasiaBank/protocol/pictures.html

For the eventcasts participants were first presented with the two sequential pictures and were asked to produce a story that was based on temporal sequencing. The tester used the following script: "*Take a little time to look at these pictures. They tell a story. Take a look at all of them, and then I'll ask you to tell me the story with a beginning, a middle, and an end. You can look at the pictures as you tell the story.*" If the participants did not respond within 10 seconds, the tester prompted them to "*Take a look at this picture* (pointing to first picture) *and tell me what you think is happening*." If needed, the tester pointed to each picture sequentially, giving the prompt: "*And what happens here?*" Subsequently participants were presented with the two single pictures and were asked to produce a story with temporal sequencing using the following script: "*Here is a picture. Look at everything that's happening and then tell me a story about what you see. Tell me the story with a beginning, a middle, and an end.*" Feedback was provided to avoid eliciting a simple description of objects, characters, and/or their physical characteristics. Participants also viewed and told the story depicted in a wordless picture book of *Cinderella*. Participants were presented with the stimulus book and were allowed as much time as they desired to view it and remind themselves of the story. Then, the book was removed and they were asked to "Tell the story in their own words".

Transcription and language sample preparation. Samples were digitally recorded and then orthographically transcribed in the CHAT format that is compatible with a set of programs called CLAN (MacWhinney, 2000). Samples were then segmented into c-units. A c-unit is a communication unit and includes an independent clause with its modifiers (Loban, 1976); it is commonly used to segment oral discourse samples (Hughes, McGillivray, & Schmidek, 1997). The following is an example of a c-unit:

Pre-c-unit segmented sample:

Oh little Sally's cat Chico got up in the tree again and daddy who is afraid of heights did his best to try to rescue him.

C-unit segmented:

(1) Oh little Sally's cat Chico got up in the tree again.

(2) And daddy who is afraid of heights did his best to try to rescue him.

Approximately 10% of the samples from each group were randomly selected and transcribed again for reliability purposes. For both groups, intra- and inter-rater word-by-word transcription reliability was above 90%.

Lexical diversity

Following segmentation, each word was tagged morphosyntactically. Because function words have little or ambiguous meaning and convey predominantly grammatical relationships, they were removed from the samples, leaving only content words (i.e., nouns, verbs, adjectives and *-ly* adverbs). Further, to avoid conflating LD with grammaticality, only unique lexical representations were counted as separate types. This was approximated by performing a lemma-based analysis of LD. To determine which affixes to retain we used Kiparsky's (1982) levels of morphological derivation. Level three inflections that do not alter the meaning of a stem were disregarded. For example, eat, eats, and ate were all considered three tokens of the same type.

Also, for both groups, repetitions, repairs, and filler words were excluded from further analysis.

Samples from PWA were further coded and all paraphasias were excluded from analysis (a) to ensure that estimates of LD reflected the efficiency of word access and retrieval as discussed within Dell and Chapelle's model (specifically, Chapelle's fourth dimension) and (b) because they distort the common code between interlocutors that is prerequisite for efficient and successful communication (Jakobson, 1971). Finally, *D* was calculated using the voc-*D* program in CLAN. The code used for the analysis can be found at www.asu.edu/clas/shs/aald/current_research.html. See MacWhinney, Fromm, Holland, Forbes, and Wright (2010) for a more detailed example of automated analyses performed using CLAN.

D has been described in detail elsewhere, and therefore only a brief review of the approach is offered here (cf. MacWhinney, 2000; McCarthy & Jarvis, 2007; McKee et al., 2000). For each language sample, calculating *D* involves a series of random text samplings to plot an empirical TTR versus number-of-tokens curve (see Figure 1). First, 35 tokens are randomly drawn from the text without replacement and the TTR is computed. This process is repeated 100 times and the average TTR for 35 tokens is estimated and plotted. The same routine is then repeated for subsamples from 36 to 50 tokens. The average TTR for each subsample of increasing token size is subsequently plotted to form the empirical curve. Then the estimation of *D* proceeds by producing a theoretical curve that maximises the fit to the empirical TTR curve using the least squares approach. Because *D* is the product of a sampling, stochastic process, its value varies each time the program is run. For that reason the whole process is repeated three times and the final *D* value is the average of the three runs.

RESULTS

Preliminary analysis

Prior to performing the statistical analyses for addressing the study aims, data were examined through various PASW Statistics 18.0.1 (SPSS Inc.) programs for accuracy of data entry, missing values, univariate outliers with extreme *z* scores (larger than 3.3), and fit between variables' distributions and the assumptions of univariate analysis

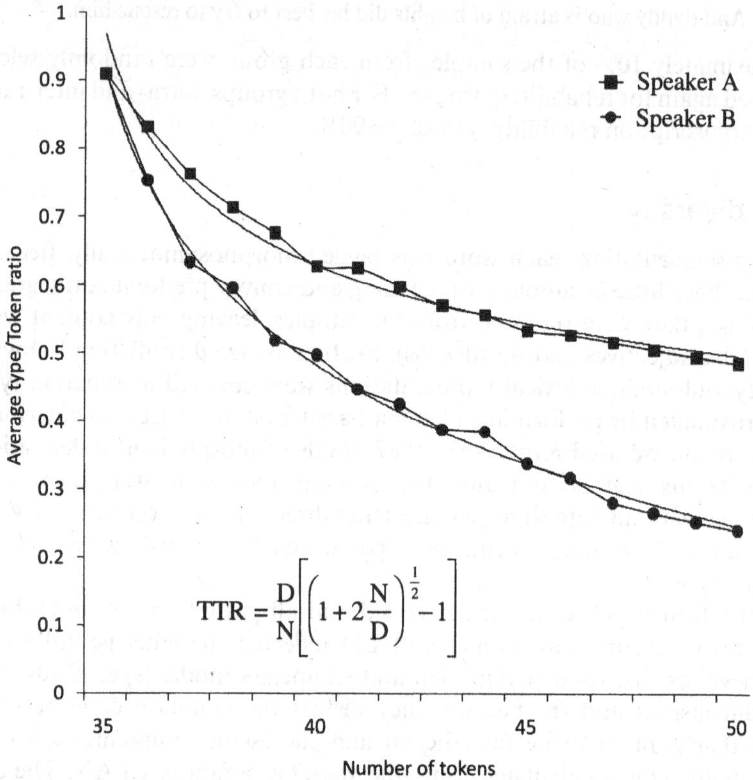

Figure 1. Estimating *D*. Average type–token ratio (TTR) decreases as a function of sample length (N) for two speakers. Speaker A uses more diverse vocabulary (i.e., uses the same words less often) and his/her average TTR decreases at a slow pace. Speaker B uses the same words repeatedly and her/his TTR decreases faster as a function of the sample size. voc-*D* captures a speaker's lexical diversity by modelling how fast the average TTR decreases. The slope of the fitted nonlinear curve corresponds to different *D* values. The steeper the slope of the fitted line, the lower the *D* value. Selection of the best-fitting curve is determined using a least squares approach.

(i.e., gross violations of normality and homoscedasticity). The data were examined separately for the two groups. No outliers were identified for either group. For the PWA, two cases had fewer than 50 tokens after function words and paraphasias were excluded from their language samples, and as a result *D* was not estimated. These cases were not included in the analysis, leaving 25 cases in the PWA group. For the NIA group no missing data were observed. The shape of the distributions of the dependent variable *D* was assessed using histograms and was found satisfactory (skewness and kurtosis ranged from –1 to +1). The assumption regarding homogeneity of variances, as assessed using Levene's test, was also met. Regarding the language samples, the average numbers of tokens across different conditions are shown in Table 2.

Lexical diversity across group and discourse task

A 2 × 3 mixed ANOVA was conducted that included group (NIA, PWA) and task (single pictures, sequential pictures, and story telling). The former was the between-participants factor and the latter the within-participants factor. Significant results

TABLE 2
Mean number of content words for each elicitation task across groups

	PWA group	*NIA group*
Single pictures	76.33 (*SD* = 10.85)	119.78 (*SD* = 9.64)
Sequential pictures	68.89 (*SD* = 6.04)	119.48 (*SD* = 8.29)
Story telling	124.15 (*SD* = 15.59)	289.40 (*SD* = 29.40)

were found for the discourse task main effect, $\Lambda = .43$, $F(2, 49) = 33.52$, $p < .01$, *partial* $\eta^2 = .57$, and the interaction, $\Lambda = .65$, $F(2, 49) = 13.42$, $p < .01$, *partial* $\eta^2 = .35$. The group main effect was also significant, $F(1, 50) = 78.23$, $p < .01$, *partial* $\eta^2 = .61$.

To better understand the significant interaction, group and discourse task simple effects were examined by conducting a series of independent sample *t*-tests and paired-sample *t*-tests, respectively. To control for Type I error, familywise alpha was set to .0125 and .025 for each age and discourse task simple main effect, respectively (Maxwell & Delaney, 2004). Subsequently, familywise error rate across the *t*-tests was controlled using the Holm's sequential Bonferroni approach.

According to the results, NIA demonstrated higher LD across all three elicitation techniques of discourse compared to PWA. For both groups, single pictures were associated with the lowest LD. However, for the NIA group, story telling yielded higher LD than the sequential pictures; whereas PWA exhibited similar LD for the story and sequential pictures (see Figure 2). All comparisons were significant with the exception of the comparison of LD between story telling and sequential pictures for PWA, $t(24) = .64$, $p = .53$ (see Tables 3 and 4).

To further investigate LD patterns across groups and task elicitation techniques, the significant interaction was further followed up with tetrad comparisons. The mean

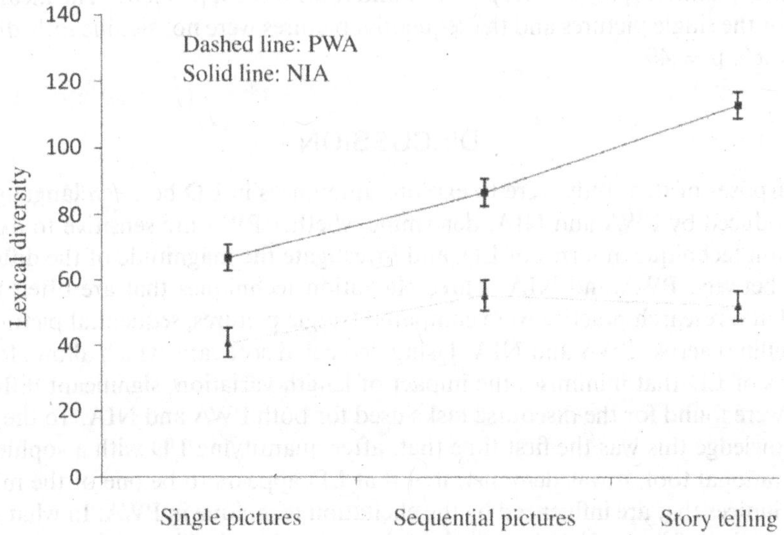

Figure 2. Mean lexical diversity for each elicitation task within each group.

TABLE 3
Mean lexical diversity scores and standard errors (SE) for PWA and NIA and group differences for each discourse elicitation task

Discourse task	*PWA group*		*NIA group*			
	M	*SE*	*M*	*SE*	*t(50)*	*p*
Single pictures	40.81	3.20	66.65	4.03	−4.96	.000*
Sequential pictures	55.10	4.33	86.48	4.17	−5.22	.000*
Story telling	52.07	4.94	112.53	4.75	−8.82	.000*

To control for Type I Error, *alpha* was set to .0125 for each simple effect.
*$p < .0125$.

TABLE 4
Mean lexical diversity differences and standard errors (SE) and comparisons among discourse elicitation task for each group

Comparison	*Mean Δ*	*SE*	*t(24)*[a]	*p*
PWA				
Single vs Sequential pictures	−14.29	4.22	−3.38	.002*
Single pictures vs Story telling	−11.26	3.91	−2.08	.008*
Sequential pictures vs Story telling	3.03	4.76	.64	.53
NIA				
Single vs Sequential pictures	−19.83	5.69	−3.49	.002*
Single pictures vs Story telling	−45.87	5.75	−7.99	.000*
Sequential pictures vs Story telling	−26.05	5.38	−4.84	.000*

To control for Type I Error, *alpha* was set to .008 for each simple effect.
[a]Paired sample *t* was conducted with 26 *df* for the NIA group.
*$p < .008$.

difference in LD for the Cinderella story was significantly larger between the two groups compared to the mean difference in LD for the single pictures as well as the sequential pictures, $t(40) = 4.42, p < .001$ and $t(40) = 3.63$, p = .001. The mean differences for the single pictures and the sequential pictures were not significantly different, $t(40) = .69$, p = .49.

DISCUSSION

The purposes of this study were to explore differences in LD between language samples produced by PWA and NIA, determine whether PWA are sensitive to discourse elicitation technique in terms of LD, and investigate the magnitude of the differences in LD between PWA and NIA. Three elicitation techniques that are often used in clinical and research practice were compared (single pictures, sequential pictures, and story telling) across PWA and NIA. Using dedicated software, which allows for comparisons of LD that minimises the impact of length variation, significant differences in LD were found for the discourse tasks used for both PWA and NIA. To the best of our knowledge this was the first time that, after quantifying LD with a sophisticated computational tool, it was demonstrated that LD appears to be one of the microlinguistic indices that are influenced by the elicitation technique in PWA. In what follows is a discussion of the results, their methodological and clinical implications, and future directions.

For the NIA, results replicate and extend previous findings in the literature (Fergadiotis et al., 2010; Wright & Capilouto, 2009). As in the aforementioned studies, in our case NIA demonstrated highest levels of LD for story telling, followed by sequential pictures; and, single pictures elicited the least lexically diverse samples. However, one limitation of the previous studies is that neither one had conducted a lemma-based analysis. We addressed this issue by utilising an analysis that excluded functions words, and considered variations of the same stem as the same type. By accounting only for content words in this way, *D* is believed to better reflect LD.

One of the main goals of the study was to establish the difference between NIA and PWA in terms of LD during discourse production. Discourse production entails the activation and interaction of multiple interconnected cognitive and linguistic subsystems that are often impaired in PWA. In our study PWA demonstrated significantly lower LD than NIA across discourse tasks. Given that the two groups were matched for age, gender, and education, it is unlikely that this finding was driven by differences in the first three dimensions of Chapelle's (1994) model. If one accepts that aphasia is caused primarily by an access deficit that affects language processing rather than loss of language per se, then our results most likely reflect the limited resources of PWA for accessing and retrieving lexical items. Specifically, limited LD may be a manifestation of (a) the erroneous responses that take the form of lexical and sublexical paraphasias (e.g., literal and semantic paraphasias), and (b) the inability to map from the conceptual representation to the phonological form that could lead to omissions and often lends itself to avoidance strategies and circumlocutions. The latter point highlights a characteristic behaviour that is more prominent to language production at the discourse level as opposed to confrontational naming. That is, when PWA anticipate or use problematic vocabulary, they may resort to more familiar words that can result in altering or simplifying their message.

Regarding the impact of discourse task on LD, PWA showed both similarities as well as differences compared to NIA. First, PWA demonstrated significantly higher LD for sequential pictures than single pictures, similarly to NIA. Capilouto, Wright, and Wagovich (2005) have suggested that sequential stimuli provide the participants with additional temporal and causal information about the depicted story. As a result, participants' verbal output in response to sequential pictures can be more lexically diverse because it attempts to convey representations that entail a larger number and/or more complex relationships between characters and events. Expressing a larger number and/or more complicated interactions would require the introduction of specific vocabulary; in turn, increasing the likelihood of sampling from a wider variety of lexical items and thus producing new vocabulary. In the absence of such additional information though (i.e., in the case of the single pictures) participants may have a higher probability to simply "list" events without considering the underlying relationships, and therefore be more prone to repetition. A relevant implication that pertains both to the clinical and research fields is that sequential pictures can be used to obtain a more diverse language sample in terms of lexical items that translates into more opportunities to observe behaviours of interest.

Further, PWA demonstrated an analogous decrease in LD for single and sequential stimuli compared to their matched controls. For these types of tasks, results of the three-tier analysis are suggestive of an undifferentiated limitation in PWAs' ability to demonstrate a range of vocabulary that would be comparable to that exhibited by NIA. In other words, the impact of aphasia in terms of LD appears to be the same regardless of whether one chooses to use single or sequential pictures to elicit the discourse samples.

However, as opposed to single and sequential pictures, when narratives were elicited using the story-telling format, PWA demonstrated a significantly larger difference (see Figure 2) compared to NIA. Whereas NIA showed evidence of higher LD for story telling compared to sequential pictures, PWA failed to demonstrate a similar pattern. Instead, PWA exhibited similar LD for story telling and sequential pictures. This finding suggests that PWA may be more susceptible to the demands associated with specific elicitation techniques (in this case story telling). Several possible and potentially inclusive explanations could be proposed to account for these results. First, the story-retelling task is performed without pictorial support during discourse generation. So, PWA have to produce a narrative without the scaffolding provided by the illustrations that may serve as a cognitive map or schema. The absence of immediate visual support may force participants to allocate more resources on memory, planning, and organisational processes. Such an account rests on the assumption that the autonomous low-level cognitive process of lexical access shares resources with higher-order cognitive processes. Some recent findings appear to be in favour of this hypothesis that nevertheless merits further investigation (Rabovsky, Álvarez, Hohlfeld, & Sommer, 2008). At the same time it possible that the illustrations are priming the semantic/conceptual content of the depicted words, thus boosting their activation and allowing them to be more easily retrieved. This account, which is consistent with spreading activation models, would suggest that tasks that lack the contextual support in the form of pictures might be harder for PWA. In addition to the theoretical significance, this finding is clinically important and should be explored further in future investigations because it suggests that story telling has a greater discriminatory potential that could be tapped for diagnostic purposes.

CONCLUSIONS

Taken as a whole, these results provide additional support for the notion that the nature of the task contributes to the cognitive and linguistic demands that are imposed on the speakers (Armstrong, 2000; Coelho, 2002; Cooper, 1990). In other words, individuals' LD performance can vary both as a function of the individual's latent trait, as well as from the discourse type that the participant chooses to produce in response to a discourse elicitation technique. A critical methodological implication is that if LD is to be explored in discourse samples produced by adults with or without neurogenic communication impairments, it might be useful to include a "type of discourse" factor in the analysis rather than collapsing or aggregating the data. Including such a factor may present an advantage because it would facilitate a more accurate modelling of the data.

One limitation of this study is that LD was quantified using a single index (i.e., *D*). By including multiple indicators (such as the measure of textual lexical diversity; McCarthy, 2005), it would be possible to use statistical methods for a richer and more accurate investigation of LD. For example, using a latent variable modelling approach, one would be able to (1) operationally define LD as an unobserved trait that characterises individuals, (2) consider their discourse as the observed manifestation that enables us to make inferences about the individuals' level of LD, and (3) obtain error-free estimates of individuals' LD. This interactionalist approach would allow researchers to put forward questions about individuals' discourse abilities by examining their language outputs. Further, if the distinction between the trait and the manifest variables is made clear, then researchers can conduct a wide variety of analyses to understand both the nature of cognitive-communicative deficits and take into account the "peculiarities" of the methods that are used to elicit language samples.

Considering that the word retrieval difficulties experienced by PWA can severely limit their participation in communicative activities and negatively affect their discourse production, indices that assess their performance at the discourse level can prove to be very informative. LD, which is quantified in this study using a method that is robust to length variation, can complement other discourse measures in an attempt to assess the impact of word finding deficits at the discourse level. The way *D* was employed in this study does not provide direct insight into the complex interactions of the linguistic systems that are involved in accessing and retrieving lexical items. However, it does allow us to construct a more detailed account of the richness of their verbal output. Future investigations using LD and measures such as story-telling propositions and information units will further enhance our understanding of how the capacity to employ a large lexicon is associated with more efficient communication; and in turn, they may lead to the development of more valid and reliable treatment outcome measures.

REFERENCES

Armstrong, E. (2000). Aphasic discourse analysis: The story so far. *Aphasiology*, *14*(9), 875–892. doi:10.1080/02687030050127685

Ash, S., Moore, P., Antani, S., McCawley, G., Work, M., & Grossman, M. (2006). Trying to tell a tale: Discourse impairments in progressive aphasia and frontotemporal dementia. *Neurology*, *66*(9), 1405–1413. doi:10.1212/01.wnl.0000210435.72614.38

Ballard, K., & Thompson, K. (1999). Treatment and generalization of complex sentence production in agrammatism. *Journal of Speech, Language, and Hearing Research*, *42*(3), 690–707.

Balota, D. A., & Chumbley, J. I. (1984). Are lexical decisions a good measure of lexical access? The role of word frequency in the neglected decision stage. *Journal of Experimental Psychology: Human Perception and Performance*, *10*(3), 340–357. doi: 10.1037/0096-1523.10.3.340

Bliss, L. S., & McCabe, A. (2006). Comparison of discourse genres: Clinical implications. *Contemporary Issues in Communication Science and Disorders*, *33*(2), 126–137.

Bock, J. K. (1982). Toward a cognitive psychology of syntax: Information processing contributions to sentence formulation. *Psychological Review*, *89*(1), 1–47.

Brady, M., Armstrong, L., & Mackenzie, C. (2005). Further evidence on topic use following right hemisphere brain damage: Procedural and descriptive discourse. *Aphasiology*, *19*(8), 731–747. doi:10.1080/02687030500141430

Brink, T. L., Yesavage, J. A., Lum, O., Heersema, P., Adey, M. B., & Rose, T.L. (1982). Screening tests for geriatric depression. *Clinical Gerontologist*, *1*, 37–44.

Brookshire, R. H., & Nicholas, L. E. (1994). Speech sample size and test–retest stability of connected speech measures for adults with aphasia. *Journal of Speech & Hearing Research*, *37*(2), 399–407.

Cameron, R. M., Wambaugh, J. L., Wright, S. M., & Nessler, C. L. (2006). Effects of a combined semantic/phonologic cueing treatment on word retrieval in discourse. *Aphasiology*, *20*(2–4), 269–285. doi:10.1080/02687030500473387

Capilouto, G., Wright, H. H., & Wagovich, S. A. (2005). CIU and main event analyses of the structured discourse of older and younger adults. *Journal of Communication Disorders*, *38*(6), 431–444. doi:10.1016/j.jcomdis.2005.03.005

Carroll, J. B. (1964). *Language and thought*. Englewood Cliffs, NJ: Prentice-Hall.

Chapelle, C. A. (1994). Are C-tests valid measures for L2 vocabulary research? *Second Language Research*, *10*(2), 157–187.

Chomsky, N. (1980). *Rules and representations*. New York, NY: Columbia University Press.

Christiansen, J. A. (1995). Coherence violations and propositional usage in the narratives of fluent aphasics. *Brain and Language*, *51*, 291–317.

Coelho, C. A. (2002). Story narratives of adults with closed head injury and non-brain-injured adults: Influence of socioeconomic status, elicitation task, and executive functioning. *Journal of Speech, Language, and Hearing Research*, *45*(6), 1232–1248. doi:10.1044/1092-4388(2002/099

Coelho, C. A., Grela, B., Corso, M., Gamble, A., & Feinn, R. (2005). Microlinguistic deficits in the narrative discourse of adults with traumatic brain injury. *Brain Injury*, *19*(13), 1139–1145. doi:10.1080/02699050500110678

Cooper, P. V. (1990). Discourse production and normal aging: Performance on oral picture description tasks. *Journals of Gerontology*, *45*(5), 210–214.

del Toro, C. M., Altmann, L. J. P., Raymer, A. M., Leon, S., Blonder, L. X., & Rothi, L. J. G. (2008). Changes in aphasic discourse after contrasting treatments for anomia. *Aphasiology*, *22*(7–8), 881–892. doi:10.1080/02687030701844204

Dell, G. G. S. (1986). A spreading-activation theory of retrieval in sentence production. *Psychological Review*, *93*(3), 283–321.

Dell, G. S., Oppenheim, G. M., & Kittredge, K. A., (2008) Saying the right word at the right time: Syntagmatic and paradigmatic interference in sentence production. *Language and cognitive processes*, *23*(4), 583–608.

Dell, G. S., Schwartz, M. F., Martin, N., Saffran, E. M., & Gagnon, D. A. (1997). Lexical access in aphasic and non-aphasic speakers. *Psychological Review*, *104* (4), 801–838.

Doyle, P. J., McNeil, M. R., Spencer, K. A., Goda, A. J., Cottrell, K., & Lustig, A. P. (1998). The effects of concurrent picture presentations on retelling of orally presented stories by adults with aphasia. *Aphasiology*, *12*, 561–574.

Engber, C. A. (1995). The relationship of lexical proficiency to the quality of ESL compositions. *Journal of Second Language Writing*, *4*(2), 139–155.

Fergadiotis, G., Wright, H. H., & Capilouto, G. (2010, May). *Productive vocabulary across discourse types.* Clinical Aphasiology Conference, Isle of Palms, SC, USA.

Fleming, V. B., & Harris, J. L. (2008). Complex discourse production in mild cognitive impairment: Detecting subtle changes. *Aphasiology*, *22*(7–8), 729–740. doi:10.1080/02687030701803762

Folstein, M. F., Folstein, S. E., & McHugh, P. R. (1975). Mini-mental state: A practical method for grading the cognitive state of patients for the clinician. *Journal of Psychiatric Research*, *12*(3), 189–198. doi:10.1016/0022-3956(75)90026-6

Gordon, J. K. (2008). Measuring the lexical semantics of picture description in aphasia. *Aphasiology*, *22*(7–8), 839–852. doi:10.1080/02687030701820063

Gordon, J. K., & Dell, G. S. (2003). Learning to divide the labor: An account of deficits in light and heavy verb production. *Cognitive Science, 27*, 1–40.

Grimes, N. (2005). *Walt Disney's Cinderella*. New York, NY: Random House.

Grosjean, F. (1980). Spoken word recognition processes and the gating paradigm. *Perception and Psychophysics*, *28*, 267–283.

Guiraud, P. (1960). *Problèmes et méthodes de la statistique linguistique*. Dordrecht, The Netherlands: D. Reidel.

Halliday, M. A. K., & Hasan, R. (1989) *Language, context, and text: aspects of language in a social-semiotic perspective*. Oxford, UK: Oxford University Press.

Heath, S. B. (1986). Taking a cross-cultural look at narratives. *Topics in Language Disorders*, *7*, 84–95.

Herdan, G. (1960). *TypeToken mathematics*. The Hague, The Netherlands: Mouton.

Honda, R., Mitachi, M., & Watamori, T. S. (1999). Production of discourse in high-functioning individuals with aphasia—with reference to performance on the Japanese CADL. *Aphasiology*, *13*(6), 475–493. doi:10.1080/026870399402037

Hough, M. S., & Barrow, I. (2003). Descriptive discourse abilities of traumatic brain-injured adults. *Aphasiology*, *17*(2), 183–191. doi:10.1080/729255221

Hughes, D., McGillivray, L., & Schmidek, M. (1997). *Guide to narrative language: Procedures for assessment*. Eau Claire, WI: Thinking Publications.

Jakobson, R. (1971). Two aspects of language and two types of aphasic disturbances. In R. Jakobson & M. Halle (Eds.), *Fundamentals of language*. The Hague, The Netherlands: Mouton.

Jarvis, S. (2002). Short texts, best-fitting curves and new measures of lexical diversity. *Language Testing*, *19*(1), 57–84.

Kempen, G. & Hoenkamp, E. (1987) An incremental procedural grammar for sentence formulation. *Cognitive Science*, 11, 201–258.

Kertesz, A. (2007). *Western aphasia battery – revised*. New York, NY: Grune & Stratton.

Kiparsky, P. (1982). From cyclic phonology to lexical phonology. In H. V. D. Hulst & N. Smith (Eds.), *The structure of phonological representations*, (pp. 131–175). Dordrecht, The Netherlands: Foris Publishing.

Kroll, J. F., & Merves, J. S. (1986). Lexical access for concrete and abstract words. *Journal of Experimental Psychology: Learning, Memory, and Cognition, 12*(1), 92–107.

Lapointe, L. L., & Horner, J. (1998). *Reading comprehension battery for aphasia*. Austin, TX: Pro-Ed.

Larfeuil, C., & Le Dorze, G. (1997). An analysis of the word-finding difficulties and of the content of the discourse of recent and chronic aphasic speakers. *Aphasiology, 11*(8), 783–811. doi:10.1080/02687039708250456

Levelt, W. J. M. (1989). *Speaking: From intention to articulation*. Cambridge, MA: MIT Press.

Levelt, W. J. M., Roelofs, A., & Meyer, A. S. (1999). A theory of lexical access in speech production. *Behavioural and Brain Science*, 22(1), 991–975.

Loban, W. D. (1976). *Language development: Kindergarten through grade twelve. NCTE committee on research* (Report No. 18). Urbana, IL: National Council of Teachers of English.

Longacre, R. E. (1996). *The grammar of discourse* (2nd ed.). New York, NY: Plenum Press.

MacWhinney, B. (2000). *The CHILDES project: Tools for analysing talk, Volume 1: Transcription format and programs* (3rd ed.). Mahwah, NJ: Lawrence Erlbaum Associates.

MacWhinney, B., Fromm, D., Holland, A., Forbes, M., & Wright, H. (2010). Automated analysis of the Cinderella story. *Aphasiology. 24*(6–8), 856–868. doi:10.1080/02687030903452632

Malvern, D. D., & Richards, B. J. (1997). A new measure of lexical diversity. In A. Ryan & A. Wray (Eds.), *Evolving models of language* (pp. 58–71). Clevedon, UK: Multilingual Matters.

Maxwell, S. E., & Delaney, H. D. (2004). *Designing experiments and analysing data: A model comparison perspective* (2nd ed.). Mahwah, NJ: Lawrence Erlbaum Associates.

McCarthy, P. M. (2005). *An assessment of the range and usefulness of lexical diversity measures and the potential of the measure of textual lexical diversity* (Doctoral Dissertation). Retrieved from ProQuest Nursing & Allied Health Source Database.

McCarthy, P. M., & Jarvis, S. (2007). Vocd: A theoretical and empirical evaluation. *Language Testing, 24*(4), 459–488. doi:10.1177/0265532207080767

McCarthy, P. M., & Jarvis, S. (2010). MTLD, vocd-D, and HD-D: A validation study of sophisticated approaches to lexical diversity assessment. *Behaviour Research Methods, 42*(2), 381–392.

McKee, G., Malvern, D., & Richards, B. (2000). Measuring vocabulary diversity using dedicated software. *Literary and Linguistic Computing, 15*(3), 323–337.

McNeil, M. R., (1997). *Clinical management of sensorimotor speech disorders*. New York, NY: Thieme Medical Publishers.

McNeil, M. R., Doyle, P. J., Fossett, T. R. D., Park, G. H., & Goda, A. J. (2001). Reliability and concurrent validity of the information unit scoring metric for the story retelling procedure. *Aphasiology, 15*(10–11), 991–1006. doi:10.1080/02687040143000348

McNeil, M. R., & Pratt, S. R. (2001). Defining aphasia: Some theoretical and clinical implications of operating from a formal definition. *Aphasiology, 15*(10), 901–911. doi:10.1080/02687040143000276

McNeil, M. R., Sung, J. E., Yang, D., Pratt, S. R., Fossett, T. R. D., Doyle, P. J., et al. (2007). Comparing connected language elicitation procedures in persons with aphasia: Concurrent validation of the Story Retell Procedure. *Aphasiology, 21*(6–8), 775–790. doi:10.1080/02687030701189980

Menn, L., Reilly, K. F., Hayashi, M., Kamio, A., Fujita, I., & Sasanuma, S. (1998). The interaction of preserved pragmatics and impaired syntax in Japanese and English aphasic speech. *Brain and Language, 61*, 183–225.

Murray, L. (2009, November). *Narrative differences among elderly with clinical depression versus early Alzheimer's*. Poster session presented at the Convention of the American Speech-Language-Hearing Association, New Orleans, LA, USA.

Nicholas, L. E., & Brookshire, R. H. (1993). A system for quantifying the informativeness and efficiency of the connected speech of adults with aphasia. *Journal of Speech & Hearing Research, 36*(2), 338–350.

Olness, G. S. (2006). Genre, verb, and coherence in picture-elicited discourse of adults with aphasia. *Aphasiology, 20*(2–4), 175–187. doi:10.1080/02687030500472710

Prins, R., & Bastiaanse, R. (2004). Analysing the spontaneous speech of aphasic speakers. *Aphasiology, 18*(12), 1075–1091. doi:10.1080/02687030444000534

Prins, R. S., Snow, C. E., & Wagenaar, E. (1978). Recovery from aphasia: Spontaneous speech versus language comprehension. *Brain and Language, 6*(2), 192–211. doi:10.1016/0093-934X(78)90058-5

Rabovskya, M., Álvarez, C. J., Hohlfeld, A., & Sommer, W. (2008). Is lexical access autonomous? Evidence from combining overlapping tasks with recording event-related brain potentials. *Brain Research*, 1222, 156–165.

Rider, J. D., Wright, H. H., Marshall, R. C., & Page, J. L. (2008). Using semantic feature analysis to improve contextual discourse in adults with aphasia. *American Journal of Speech-Language Pathology, 17*(2), 161–172. doi:10.1044/1058-0360(2008/016)

Rubin, C., & Newton, E. (2001). *Capture the moment: The Pulitzer Prize photographs*. New York, NY: W. W. Norton.

Schwartz, M. F., Dell, G. S., Martin, N., Gahl, S., & Sobel, P. (2006). A case-series test of the interactive two-step model of lexical access: Evidence from picture naming. *Journal of Memory and Language*, 54, 228–264.

Tweedie, F. J., & Baayen, R. H. (1998). How variable may a constant be? Measures of lexical richness in perspective. *Computers and the Humanities*, *32*(5), 323–352.

Tyler, L. K., & Wessels, J. (1983). Quantifying contextual contributions to word recognition processes. *Perception and Psychophysics*, 34, 409–420.

Ulatowska, H. K., Allard, L., & Bond Chapman, S. (1990). Narrative and procedural discourse in aphasia. In Y. Joanette & H. H. Brownell (Eds.), *Discourse ability and brain damage: Theoretical and empirical perspectives* (pp. 180–198). New York, NY: Springer-Verlag.

Ulatowska, H. K., North, A. J., & Macaluso-Haynes, S. (1981). Production of narrative and procedural discourse in aphasia. *Brain and Language*, *13*(2), 345–371. doi:10.1016/0093-934X(81)90100-0

Vermeer, A. (2000). Coming to grips with lexical richness in spontaneous speech data. *Language Testing*, *17*(1), 65–83. doi:10.1191/026553200676636328

Wachal, R. S., & Spreen, O. (1973). Some measures of lexical diversity in aphasic and normal language performance. *Language and Speech*, *16*(2), 169–181.

Wright, H. H., & Capilouto, G. J. (2009). Manipulating task instructions to change narrative discourse performance. *Aphasiology*, *23*(10), 1295–1308. doi:10.1080/02687030902826844

Wright, H. H., & Capilouto, G. J. (2011). *Measuring age-related changes in discourse production*. Unpublished raw data.

Wright, H. H., Silverman, S. W., & Newhoff, M. (2003). Measures of lexical diversity in aphasia. *Aphasiology*, *17*(5), 443–452. doi:10.1080/02687030344000166

APHASIOLOGY, 2011, 25 (11), 1431–1447

"Better but no cigar": Persons with aphasia speak about their speech

Davida Fromm[1], Audrey Holland[2], Elizabeth Armstrong[3], Margaret Forbes[1], Brian MacWhinney[1], Amy Risko[1], and Nicole Mattison[4]

[1]Department of Psychology, Carnegie Mellon University, Pittsburgh, PA, USA
[2]University of Arizona, Tucson, AZ, USA
[3]Edith Cowan University, Joondalup, Western Australia
[4]Department of Statistics, Carnegie Mellon University, Pittsburgh, PA, USA

Background: This study examined responses of persons with aphasia (PWAs) to a general question about their speech. *Aims*: The goal was to describe their evaluative responses as positive, negative, or neutral/mixed and determine if responses differed, based on time post-onset, aphasia severity, and aphasia type.
Methods & Procedures: A total of 71 participants from the AphasiaBank project were included. As part of a larger protocol, investigators asked, "How do you think your speech is these days?" Responses were videotaped and transcribed using CLAN. Two authors coded the evaluative responses and categorised themes in the elaborative content provided by the participants.
Outcomes & Results: Positive responses accounted for 59% of all responses, followed by neutral/mixed (18%), and negative (17%). Participants also mentioned specific speech problems (35%), improvement (31%), and therapy (8%) in their responses. Time post-onset and aphasia type were not significantly associated with nature of response. Aphasia severity was significantly associated with nature of response, with higher AQ scores in the positive group and vice versa.
Conclusions: The responses are discussed in the context of self-image and self-expression in PWA and social models in aphasia therapy. Results are also compared with those of others with chronic disabilities and research on resilience, positive affect, and optimism.

Keywords: Aphasia; Personal narrative; Self-evaluation; Positive; AphasiaBank.

The increasing focus on discourse in aphasiology research attests to the fact that connected speech samples across a variety of contexts reveal important information about the aphasic speaker's linguistic and cognitive abilities, personal and social insights related to identity, adjustment to aphasia, and interactional skills (Hinckley, 2006; Shadden & Hagstrom, 2007; Simmons-Mackie & Damico, 2009). To date,

Address correspondence to: Davida Fromm PhD, Carnegie Mellon University, Department of Psychology, 5000 Forbes Avenue, Pittsburgh, PA 15213, USA. E-mail: fromm@andrew.cmu.edu
This project is funded by NIH_NIDCD grant R01-DC008524 (2007–2012). A visiting Fellowship provided by Edith Cowan University, Western Australia, to Audrey Holland resulted in Beth Armstrong's collaboration in this work.

http://dx.doi.org/10.1080/02687038.2011.608839

discourse samples used in aphasia research have included both monologic recounts of significant events in the person's life and dialogues about everyday activities and interests. Examples of such monologues include recounts of (1) frightening events (Behrns, Wengelin, Broberg, & Hartelius, 2009; Olness, Matteson, & Stewart, 2010; Ulatowska & Olness, 2001, 2003); (2) positive events such as a wedding or holiday (Armstrong, 2001); and (3) illness, particularly related to stroke stories (Armstrong & Ulatowska, 2007; Hinckley, 2006; Ulatowska, Olness, Keebler, & Tillery, 2006). Dialogic interactions have covered a variety of topics and occur in contexts such as aphasia groups or private homes (Beeke, Wilkinson, & Maxim, 2009; Oeschlager & Thorne, 1999; Simmons-Mackie & Damico, 2009). Nonetheless, by far the majority of work in aphasic discourse (in both research and clinical practice) tends to look at discourse involving picture descriptions, story retell, and procedural discourse. These all involve third-person-focused language dealing with almost anything but the life experiences of persons with aphasia (PWAs), topics familiar or interesting to them, or their (possibly emotionally tinged) attitudes.

Interest in including relevant personal experience in clinical and research discourse sampling methods parallels the emergence of social models for aphasia, which have gained traction in aphasia assessment and treatment in the last 10 years (Byng & Duchan, 2005; Elman, 2005; Simmons-Mackie et al., 2007). Stemming from such models there has been increasing advocacy to empower PWAs to play a role in the management of their own disorders and to equalise the social relations involved in service delivery. Empowerment includes altering the interactions between clinician/investigator and client/participant by asking genuine, information-seeking questions of PWAs regarding their speech, their strokes, and their recoveries. In this way, parity in clinical conversations can be restored.

Several researchers (e.g., Hagstrom, 2004; Holland, 2007; Pound, Parr, Lindsay, & Woolf, 2000; Shadden, Hagstrom, & Koski, 2008) have investigated the telling of personal stroke narratives in aphasia therapy situations and have discussed the benefits of such narratives. All agree that narratives present people with aphasia (similar to other individuals suffering from a chronic illness) with an opportunity to talk about their problems and, thereby, help to re-establish a more positive sense of self and diminish what Shadden (2005) called "identity theft". The role of the speech-language pathologist in this context is that of an active listener, "co-constructing clinical interactions in such a way as to create authentic relationships aimed at effecting relevant change" (Simmons-Mackie & Damico, 2010, p. 52).

Talking about one's own speech and language is a notion related to the healing power of personal narrative (Hinckley, 2006; Shadden & Hagstrom, 2007). Reporting on scripts developed by aphasic speakers or used in script training (Cherney, Halper, Holland, & Cole, 2008; Youmans, Holland, Munoz, & Bourgeois, 2005; Youmans, Youmans, & Hancock, 2011), Holland, Halper, and Cherney (2010) described the content of 28 self-determined monologues written and subsequently learned by persons with chronic aphasia. Of these monologues, 19 (68%) were stories about some aspect of the speaker's life and 12 (43%) were specifically about their strokes. These scripts were affirmative and optimistic, supporting the notion that, despite aphasia, many persons with chronic aphasia have NOT lost (or perhaps have re-established) their sense of identity over time.

This issue, in turn, relates to the importance of helping an aphasic individual either to capitalise on or to develop some resilience, defined here simply as the ability to bounce back from aphasia. Evidence from aphasic narratives (Hinckley, 2006) and from clinical encounters (Holland, 2010) indicates that resilience matters. This should not be surprising when one considers the rich literature relating to the palliative, if not curative effects of resilience, optimism, and positive affect in other illnesses (Edward & Warelow, 2005; Pressman & Cohen, 2005; Rasmussen, Scheier, & Greenhouse, 2009). It is likely that resilience, optimism, and identity issues change over time for PWAs, altering their attitudes towards a variety of activities and opportunities, including aphasia treatment. Although neither Holland (2010) nor Hinckley (2006) specifically analysed the effects of aphasia severity or type, Hinckley did emphasise that readjustment after aphasia takes many years.

Code and Hermann (2003) reviewed a number of factors in aphasia as they relate to emotional and psychosocial status and made a strong case for better therapeutic outcomes in people with positive mood states. Regarding time post-onset, they explained that depression is not uncommon in PWAs, citing statistics of 16% at 12 months and 29% at 2–3 years following stroke. Additionally they described how site of lesion, specifically left hemisphere frontal damage, is associated with higher frequency and severity of depression in the acute period, but cognitive and physical impairment becomes almost as important as time post-onset increases. A recent study by Hilari et al. (2010) further explored the relationship of different variables to psychological distress in the first 6 months after stroke. At 3 months post-onset, aphasia was significantly associated with psychological distress, but aphasia was not a predictor of distress at any time. They reported a complex interaction between physical, linguistic, and social variables over time.

The correspondence between site of lesion and type of aphasia would suggest the likelihood of a relationship between type of aphasia and emotional status as well. It is also intuitive to expect that participants who have marked production difficulties along with acute awareness of their deficits because of relatively good comprehension and monitoring (e.g., Broca and conduction) would experience ongoing frustration that would produce negative affect. In fact, Robinson and Benson (1981) found depression to be common (almost 50%) in a group of inpatients with chronic aphasia, and reported greater frequency and severity in patients with nonfluent aphasias compared to those with fluent or global aphasias. They used two self-rating scales and two rating scales completed by professionals. Fromm, Holland, and Swindell (1984) found depression in almost half (48%) of a group of left hemisphere stroke patients with aphasia during the first year post-onset using a self-report inventory administered by examiners. A significant correlation was found between severity of aphasia and depression; type of aphasia revealed no significant correlation. Several studies have shown that aphasia severity also has an effect on quality of life or QOL (Bose, McHugh, Schollenberger, & Buchanan, 2009; Cruice, Worrall, Hickson, & Murison, 2003; Hilari & Byng, 2009; Hilari, Wiggins, Roy, Byng, & Smith, 2003). Although the current study is more narrowly focused on direct communication to elicit personal evaluations about speech in a group of non-hospitalised people with chronic aphasia, these findings on depression and QOL suggest that time post-onset, severity, and aphasia type may play important roles in emotional valence.

Recent work exploring the language of attitudes, feelings, and opinions suggests that evaluative language, a crucial part of expression of identity, may be relatively well retained in aphasia (Armstrong, 2001; Armstrong & Ulatowska, 2007; Ferguson, Worrall, Davidson, Hersh, & Sherratt, 2010; Olness et al., 2010; Ulatowska et al., 2006). Evaluations occur on a continuum of valence from negative to positive, and can involve different types of meanings including personal affect (e.g., *I hated my time in the hospital, I loved seeing my family)*, judgement (e.g., *my speech was bad, it's now excellent*), and appreciation (e.g., *the bed was uncomfortable, the stay was too long*) (for full overview, see Martin & White, 2005). Armstrong and Ulatowska (2007) analysed stroke stories produced by participants with mild to moderately severe aphasia and examined a number of evaluative devices (the use of repetition for emphasis, direct speech, metaphoric language, and the use of emotive words and phrases). Results showed that participants were able to use evaluative language to express their attitudes and feelings in spite of their incomplete utterances and impaired syntax and semantics. Additionally, studies focusing specifically on verbal pragmatics, for example, have found that speakers with left hemisphere damage and aphasia varying both in type (nonfluent, fluent, mixed) and severity (mild, mild-moderate, moderate, moderate-severe) produce more elaborate discourse when discussing emotional vs non-emotional topics (Bloom, Borod, Obler, & Koff, 1990; Bloom, Borod, Obler, & Gerstman, 1993; Borod et al., 2000). Hence, from both identity and language performance perspectives, it may in fact be therapeutic to include personal and evaluative topics and tasks in assessment and treatment contexts.

Few studies have explored personal and evaluative discourse in large groups of PWAs and systematically evaluated the effects of time post-onset, aphasia severity, or aphasia type. As part of AphasiaBank, a project designed to create a shared database of multi-media interactions for the study of communication in aphasia, a protocol was developed to elicit various types of discourse, some of which is essentially evaluative in nature.[1] The first free speech probe in the protocol is "How do you think your speech is these days?" Based on its open-ended nature, this opening question achieved several goals. First, it starts off the interaction by valuing *the participant's* opinion on this meaningful and relevant topic. Second, it allows PWAs the opportunity to give their own assessment of their communication skills in any way they can. Third, it creates a shared perspective for the investigator and the participant as they move through the rest of the tasks. Analysis of data from this interaction can provide some indication of PWAs' ability to use evaluative language to express opinions and attitudes; it can allow us to judge the positive/negative nature or "valence" of their feelings about their speech at a particular time post-onset. In addition, by looking at the further elaborations that PWAs provide, we can derive further detail regarding their approaches and attitudes towards recovery from and adaptation to aphasia.

In describing ways for physicians to solicit patients' concerns, Robinson (2006) explains that, "in mundane conversation, as well as in physician-patient visits, the question *How are you feeling?* performs the action of soliciting an evaluation of a particular, recipient-owned, currently experienced condition that is known about by the speaker and typically related to physical health" (p. 33). Hence, the similar elicitation technique used in AphasiaBank resonates with everyday clinical practice and provides a question aimed at eliciting evaluative discourse.

Emotions and attitudes are conveyed in numerous non-verbal and paralinguistic ways, as well as through direct linguistic output (Camras, Holland, & Patterson, 1993; Pittam & Scherer, 1993). Facial expression, body language, gestures, stress patterns and intonation, loudness, speech rate, sighs, and laughs all convey important meanings. The multi-media aspect of the AphasiaBank project allows for analysis of

[1] Another article in this special issue by MacWhinney, Fromm, Forbes, and Holland discusses the entire AphasiaBank protocol in more detail and explains how to use computerised transcription and language analysis programs to study phonological, lexical, morphosyntactic, and gestural aspects of the database.

verbal and nonverbal aspects of participants' responses. However, while the nonverbal and paralinguistic aspects of the interactions elicited in this study were examined in terms of the way they supported the verbal expression of participants, this initial study focuses primarily on the verbal meanings conveyed, leaving the more detailed analysis of these other aspects to future studies. The complexity of the verbal aspects alone involved in evaluative meanings has been acknowledged (Hunston & Thompson, 2003; Martin & White, 2005). Thus the goal was to conduct a preliminary study with data from a large number and wide range of participants to explore the effects of clinical variables on emotional expression. Specifically, the following questions will be addressed:

1. What is the valence (positive, negative, neutral/mixed) of the participants' evaluative responses as expressed primarily through their verbal behaviours?
2. Is the valence of their evaluative responses associated with time post-onset, severity of aphasia, or type of aphasia?
3. What additional elaborations do participants include when answering this simple question?

METHOD

This descriptive study was conducted on one segment of a larger dataset from the AphasiaBank project. Participants, materials, and procedures from the larger project are presented and followed by an explanation of the coding and statistical analyses specific to this investigation.

AphasiaBank: Participants

The data presented here comprise the responses made by the first 71 PWAs entered into the AphasiaBank database who met the following selection criteria: (1) aphasia resulting from stroke, verified through neuroimaging and/or a clear medical diagnosis; (2) auditory and visual abilities adequate for testing; and (3) English spoken as the primary language. Co-existing apraxia and dysarthria were not exclusionary criteria, but participants with dementia or with comorbidities associated with serious cognitive consequences were excluded. The AphasiaBank project received the required IRB approval. All participants (and/or their representatives) signed consent forms for the testing and data collection, and gave approval for the data to be available for research and teaching purposes. Participants ranged in age from 35.9 to 90.7 years (mean = 64.5) and came from eight different test sites in the United States. The sample included 27 females and 44 males; 58 were right handed; 6 were left-handed; 2 were ambidextrous; and the handedness of the other 5 was unavailable. Education ranged from 12 to 25 years (mean = 15.9) and time post onset ranged from 0.5 to 39.2 years (mean = 7.4). Side of lesion was left hemisphere in 58 cases, right hemisphere in 3 cases, and unavailable in 10 cases. WAB Aphasia Quotients (AQs) ranged from 20.3 to 97.6 points (mean = 68.7). Table 1 provides a list of aphasia types based on WAB AQ subtest scores.

TABLE 1
WAB data

Aphasia types	*Frequency*
Anomic	21
Broca	16
Conduction	13
Global	2
Transcortical motor	5
Transcortical sensory	1
Wernicke	7
Not aphasic (scored above cutoff)	5
Unavailable	1

AphasiaBank: Materials and procedures

All AphasiaBank testing sessions were conducted by a licensed speech-language pathologist (SLP) or by an SLP graduate student. In most cases the investigator did not know the participant prior to the session. Testing typically took place in a room at a clinic or an aphasia centre, with the investigator and the participant seated together at a table. Often a third person was in the room to monitor the video recording. In two cases testing took place in the participant's home.

The AphasiaBank research protocol begins with the investigator saying, "I am going to be asking you to do some talking." This comment is immediately followed by the first prompt, "How do you think your speech is these days?" The prompt is delivered in a natural, conversational manner. The investigator does minimal verbal prompting, but is an attentive, active listener, providing extensive nonverbal encouragers as well as plenty of time for the participant to give as complete a response as he/she desires. This approach allows the PWA to respond in a spontaneous, open-ended fashion, and to determine what constitutes an adequate answer to the question. The goal of the investigator is to create an atmosphere that encourages the participant to provide complete responses, rather than short, interrogation-style answers. Using this simple, but uniform, technique allowed for the collection of a large number of comparable samples from different sites, by different investigators, and with different participants.

The opening prompt is followed by prompts for personal narratives, picture descriptions, story telling, and procedural discourse. Finally, a few short formal assessments of naming and repetition are completed. Aphasia Quotients from the Western Aphasia Battery Revised (WAB; Kertesz, 2007) are available for all participants.

All AphasiaBank test sessions are videotaped. Trained research assistants transcribe the discourse sections using the CHAT transcription format of the CLAN program (MacWhinney, 2000).[2] Following the guidelines set by Berndt, Wayland, Rochon, Saffran, and Schwartz, (2000), utterances are segmented based on the following hierarchy of indices: syntax, intonation, pause, semantics. Two SLPs,

[2]The movies, transcripts, and protocols are available to AphasiaBank members on the AphasiaBank website at http://talkbank.org/AphasiaBank. To apply for membership in AphasiaBank, please consult the instructions on that page.

with aphasia experience and transcription training, checked the accuracy of each transcription and the two reached forced choice agreement on all features of the transcription.

Evaluative response coding

For this study, responses to the first free speech question (*How do you think your speech is these days*?) were extracted from each transcript. CHAT transcripts include all spoken output as well as gesture coding (e.g., thumbs up, head shake) and paralinguistic events (e.g., sighs, laughs). These responses were reviewed to determine the overall evaluative response by assigning each to one of these three categories: positive, negative, or neutral/mixed. In cases where the words did not indicate a clearly positive (e.g., *great*), negative (e.g., *terrible*), or neutral/mixed (e.g., *fair*, *good*, and *bad*) response, the investigators played the videos to listen to the intonation and see the nonverbal cues (e.g., facial expressions, hand gestures, body language). For example, if a participant said that his speech is "seventy percent", it would be difficult to code that response as positive or negative from the words alone. If he said it with a smile, a thumbs-up sign, and/or a sense of pride and satisfaction, it was coded as a positive assessment. If he said it with a headshake, a thumbs-down sign, a discouraging tone of voice, and/or a frown, it was tallied as negative. If he said it with a shrug and flat intonation, it was coded neutral. Two of the authors, both native speakers of English, used these guidelines and native speaker intuition to independently code the evaluative response. Inter-rater coding agreement was 97%.

Responses were also examined for further elaborative content. One member of the research team identified three themes frequently included by respondents, and a second researcher independently corroborated those findings. Then two other members of the research team independently categorised these responses into one of the three response types. Inter-rater agreement was 99% for this categorisation of the elaborative comments.

Statistical analysis

Descriptive statistics (measures of central tendency and measurement variability for interval data; tallies of frequency of occurrence for categorical data) were used in conjunction with planned inferential statistics. In particular, a two-tailed Welch's t-test (no assumption of equal population variances) was used to analyse differences between the positive and negative response groups in time post-onset and aphasia severity. Pearson's Chi-square test, the standard analysis for categorical data, was used to analyse the association between aphasia type (as categorised by WAB) and evaluative response category (positive, negative, or neutral/mixed).

RESULTS

In response to the prompt, the average number of utterances, including incomplete ones, was 4.63 (range = 1–26, $SD = 4.28$). The average number of words used in the responses (excluding word repetitions, fillers, and revisions) was 23.23 (range = 1–162, $SD = 27.17$).

Evaluative response

Responses were grouped into three categories, which accounted for 94% of all responses. The remaining 6% were removed from the main categorical analysis because they were uninterpretable, incoherent utterances often with neologisms and paraphasias (e.g., "It, it usually depends upon how long I, how long I get, I get *grags*. I get, I get, I just have to make my one *tek* in the *teks*. One, one a *teks*. But that, that, that's about it."). The three main categories as well as their corresponding percentages, definitions, and examples are given below:

1. *Positive* responses (59%) were those in which the verbal and nonverbal communication indicated a favourable assessment.
2. *Negative* responses (17%) were those in which the verbal and nonverbal communication reflected an unfavourable assessment.
3. *Neutral/mixed* responses (18%) indicated a noncommittal, average, or mixed assessment.

Positive responses mentioned improvement, getting better, and words like *fine*, *good*, *pretty good*, *really good*, *great*, *normal*, and *excellent*. Negative responses described not being able to talk and having trouble. They included words like *awful*, *terrible*, *not good*, *not well*, and *none*. Neutral/mixed responses were characterised by words such as *average* and *fair*. This category also had elements of mixed positive and negative assessments, indicating that sometimes speech is good but sometimes it is not.

Table 2 includes examples of responses from each of these categories. Paraphasias and neologisms appear in italics. Although gestures and paralinguistic behaviours are indicated in these transcription excerpts, a cautionary note is offered for reading the response examples without the benefit of actually seeing and hearing the facial expressions, gestures, body language, and vocal intonation that characterised the responses. All extra-linguistic phenomena were taken into consideration by the coders at the time of coding (native English speakers using native speaker intuition), even though these phenomena are not fully represented in the transcripts.

Associations among variables

Box plots (Tukey, 1977), shown in Figure 1, were constructed to examine the relationship between time post-onset and category of evaluative response: positive (1) versus negative (2) versus neutral/mixed (3). The dark-black vertical lines inside the boxes indicate the median time post-onset for each of the response categories, the outside edges of the boxes indicate the first and third quartiles, and the vertical lines on either end of the dashed lines indicate the lower and upper extreme non-outlier values of time post-onset. The open circles indicate outlier values because they are more than 1.5 times the inter-quartile range (difference between the first and third quartiles). The positive (1), negative (2), and neutral/mixed (3) response distributions can clearly be seen as overlapping, so no further statistical analyses were conducted on the time post-onset variable.

Box plots were also constructed to examine the relationship between the WAB Aphasia Quotient (AQ), as a measure of aphasia severity, and positive (1) versus negative (2) responses. Figure 2 shows the box plots, which suggest a difference in category

TABLE 2
Examples of responses from participants by valence rating

Rating	*Participant response*
Positive	Really good from the uh oh stroke.
	Talking better now.
	Well it's better than it used to *bid*.
	It's little bit *begger*.
	Improving, improving. I uh *cofidlitly* improving a lot better.
	Well excellent because I have had aphasia.
	Seventy, eighty percent.
	Now pretty darn good.
	Good. I'm great (gestures: thumbs up).
	I think it's normal.
	(gestures: counts) one, two, three, four, five, six, seven, eight, nine, ninety percent.
	Well, better but no cigar.
	Fine.
	Uh, uh, uh, well, uh, uh, uh, uh, uh, uh, uh, uh, uh, uh I could &uh I could talk, you know.
Negative	Not good. I'm not good at this.
	I can't talk.
	Not so well.
	No.
	Oh it's awful.
	It is terrible. It's just terrible. It was, because I can't, uh it was, I was, I . . . Oh Jesus. I, I'm so *dadut* and then boom. Buh, buh, buh, buh, buh, buh. None, none, none, none, none.
	I think it's pretty awful then. I mean it used to be pretty good but now I have trouble doing some of this.
Neutral/Mixed	Uh, fair.
	Sometime words yes, no (gestures: fair).
	Not bad. I don't know how good it is but it's not bad.
	Just not too good but improving.
	Uh well I would say is below average. In fact sub sub below average (laughs). But when you, you uh uh if you compare my speech versus another, another patient, is on par.
	Average. You know, I get most of it but I have a, I, most of it's all pretty well tire also.
	It varies. Um I'm usually good in the morning and in the afternoon. By that time I get um not uh sloppy. Not sloppy but I'm tired. And that determines how I do.

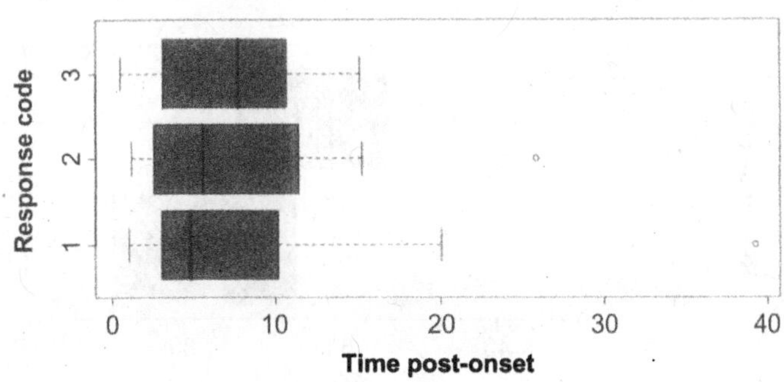

Figure 1. Boxplots of time post-onset (in years) for positive (code 1, $n = 42$) vs negative (code 2, $n = 12$) vs neutral/mixed (code 3, $n = 13$) response valence.

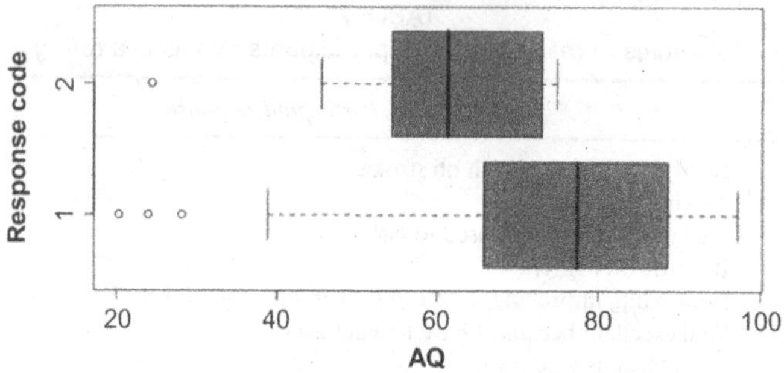

Figure 2. Boxplots of WAB AQ for positive (code 1, $n = 42$) vs negative (code 2, $n = 12$) response valence.

of evaluative response as a function of severity. The positive response group is shifted higher on the x-axis, indicating higher AQ scores (lower aphasia severity). As the figure shows, the median score for the positive response group is higher on the AQ scale than the upper extreme value for the negative response group. It is also apparent that the distribution for the positive response group is negatively skewed, indicating more positive responses in the higher AQ range. In contrast, the negative response distribution is positively skewed, indicating more negative responses in the lower AQ range. A Welch Two Sample two-tailed *t*-test showed that the difference between these two distributions was significant, $t(24.83) = 2.55$, $p = .017$. This significant difference was maintained when neutral/mixed responses were added to the positive group, thereby creating a "not negative" response group to compare with the negative response group, $t(20.79) = 2.84$, $p = .010$. Figure 3 shows the box plots for this comparison, which is similar to the previous one.

To examine the relationship between evaluative response category (positive, negative, neutral/mixed) and type of aphasia, Pearson's Chi-square test was used. For type of aphasia, the groups were Anomic, Broca, Conduction, and Wernicke. The sample sizes for other types of aphasia were too small (five or fewer) to permit their inclusion in the chi-square analysis. Results showed no significant relationship, $\chi^2(6) = 9.68$, $p = .138$, between response content and aphasia type.

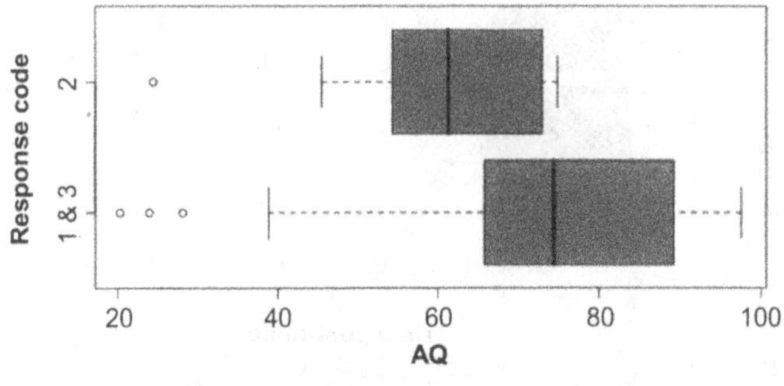

Figure 3. Boxplot of WAB AQ for positive and neutral/mixed (codes 1&3, $n = 55$) vs negative (code 2, $n = 12$) response valence.

Specific content

In addition to giving general qualitative assessments (e.g., good, bad, fair), many participants spontaneously elaborated about their speech with content that could be classified into these three topic areas: specific speech problems ($n = 25$), improvement ($n = 22$), and therapy ($n = 6$).

1. *Specific problems* included any mention of examples of their speech problems, such as getting stuck and having words spinning around in the head, speaking slowly, not rushing, not being able to talk at all, and needing to work on reading.
2. *Improvement* included any mention of positive change over time. For instance, participants mentioned getting better, improving, and being clearer.
3. *Therapy* included any mention of any kind of treatment or outside help. These utterances included speech therapy, group therapy, acupuncture treatment, and the internet.
4. Examples of responses from each of these categories appear in Table 3.

TABLE 3
Examples of specific elaborated content by content category

Category	*Participant response*
Specific speech problems	If I don't rush what I'm trying to say I could get my words across pretty well.
	It's, it's good but it's very slow. It's (gestures: no) not, not, not when I talk fast but when I talk slow I understand better.
	Sometimes I do get like stuck when I'm like trying to say something and it doesn't come out. Like I have words that are (gestures: spin) spinning around in my head. And I'm (gestures: pick) like trying to pick out which one I should say first.
	But I can't (points: mouth), it, I, you know takes me quite a long time with aphasia.
	I got a long ways to go for reading. But that's one of the most important thing for me is, is to read.
	I remember I couldn't talk at all. Thirty one days of saying ______, my name. And now talk too too much.
Improvement	My speech is fine. Um slowly it's improving.
	Not bad. Much better than a year ago.
	Better and better and better and better.
	Getting better. Getting better.
	Much better. During the stroke, well after the stroke, I couldn't talk at all. So, it's much better. Much better.
	A little bit clearer in the words.
	Better. Little bit better.
	Compared to what? I'll compare it to a year ago. I think it's a little bit better. Compared to when I first had my stroke it's A- number-one (laughs). Because when I first had my stroke I couldn't speak.
Therapy	I go to school for speech (gestures: four) two, three, four years.
	And I got into a group of people from, uh people who were *helling* me with um uh speaking.
	Uh, *entapucture*. Saturday, each Saturday. Uh needles, needles.
	The (points: here) I like. One, two (gestures: two) days is (points: here). And the internet (points: computer). I one (points: self).
	One two (points: up). I one uh a big one (gestures: big).

DISCUSSION

When asked about their speech, 59% of the PWAs gave distinctly positive answers. Another 18% of the answers were categorised as neutral/mixed. Only 17% of the participants gave negative responses to the question. The favourable spin may seem surprising in light of the chronic language impairments that most of these individuals experience. It does, however, correspond to the affirmative and optimistic descriptions of aphasic narratives and monologic scripts (Cherney et al., 2008; Hinckley, 2006). While the reasons for the optimism can be explored further, the simple fact of its existence is noteworthy as well as potentially beneficial for the participants and useful for clinicians.

Time post-onset and type of aphasia were not significantly related to positive versus negative responses. However, aphasia severity (as measured by WAB AQ) was significantly related, with higher AQ scores in the positive response group and lower AQ scores in the group with negative responses. Even when the neutral/mixed responses were combined with the positive response group to create a "not negative" response group to compare with the negative response group, the difference was still significant.

These results suggest that these PWAs are responding in what appears to be a realistic way to their situations. Those whose language is more impaired are, in fact, saying more negative things about their speech, and vice versa. In a review of positive affect and health, Pressman and Cohen (2005) described this type of relationship, namely that positive affect declines with increases in disease severity. The fact that type of aphasia was equally distributed across the positive and negative response groups suggests that the specific pattern of impairment and corresponding brain lesions had no effect on the individual's expressed opinion of his/her speech. That being said, not all types of aphasia were included in this analysis as the sample sizes were too small for transcortical sensory, transcortical motor, global aphasia, and not-aphasic-by-WAB (scored above the AQ cutoff but considered themselves aphasic). Results on the time post-onset variable may have been different if the study had been done using a longitudinal design or if participants had incurred their strokes more recently or were less well served professionally. The average time post-onset in this study was over 7 years, so this was predominantly a group of people who had been living with aphasia for a while, having been involved in speech-language therapy and stroke groups to varying extents.

The large percentage of positive responses may be due to a number of factors. One possible explanation is that, in general, people are naturally inclined towards optimism rather than pessimism. Similarly, it could be that PWAs who participate in research projects are a self-selected group with a more positive attitude. (To the authors' knowledge this factor has not been well studied in the research literature.) Not only did individuals in this study agree to participate in a study that involved sharing their language problems with researchers and students in a very direct (though identity-protected) way, the majority of them (73%) participate in aphasia centres and programmes designed to implement Life Participation Approaches to living with chronic aphasia (Chapey et al., 2000). The predominant attitudes expressed in this investigation reflect those that such centres and programmes foster and support.

One might imagine that these positive responses may simply be a case of phatic communication, much like when people say *good* or *fine* in response to standard *how are you* queries. However, the responses we obtained to this probe typically involved multiple utterances that went beyond the requirements of a minimal phatic response.

Of course, even these extended responses to this question could be viewed as constrained by further discourse expectations. For example, Button and Casey (1985) characterised the responses to *How are you* questions as "itemised news inquiries". Such responses may minimise negative evaluations. More generally, there is a preference (Pomerantz, 1984) for positive responses to questions over negative responses. It is possible that this preference is further amplified within the context of institutional discourse. However, the analyses of doctor–patient communication presented by Heritage and Clayman (2010) suggest that these communications are typically fairly frank and direct, because it is not in the patient's interest to misrepresent his or her medical and emotional status.

The actual shape of the probe we used was designed to minimise superficial or phatic responses to the question. In this regard, Robinson (2006) contrasts the *How are you?* question with the *How are you feeling?* question and explains that the former asks for a person's current and general state of being, whereas the latter requests an evaluation of the "state of a particular and ongoing health condition" (p. 39). The former question is more likely to produce a response like "*Okay*". In the current study the prompt of *How do you think your speech is these days*? led a majority of the participants to elaborate on their responses, however briefly. Also, it is worth emphasising that this question was not posed casually. The investigator poses it in a serious, deliberate manner to initiate the AphasiaBank protocol. This can be verified directly by playing back interactions directly over the web using the interactive browser facility at http://talkbank.org.

Finally, the possibility exists that there is good cause for optimism, given the fact that, in most cases, participants have improved since they first had their strokes. Improvement was specifically mentioned in many of the positive responses. Along these same lines, Riis et al. (2005) found that healthy people tend to underestimate the self-reported wellbeing of people with chronic disabilities. In studying patients with chronic kidney disease on haemodialysis, the authors found that patients adapt to their conditions and report positive average moods that do not differ significantly from those of healthy controls. The authors conclude that, in coping with hardship, patients may focus more on positive experience as an important part of their adaptation process. Similarly, Cruice, Worrall, Hickson, and Murison (2009) compared quality of life assessments from 30 people with aphasia to the assessments provided by their spouses and children, concluding that significant others rated their partners' global and health-related quality of life much lower than their aphasic partners rated themselves. While the current study does not purport to be a measure of quality of life, the positive responses by people with aphasia to a question about their speech status fit with the generally more positive ratings given by aphasic participants in these quality of life studies.

Cranfill and Wright (2010) examined quality of life measures with the goal of determining which domains are important to persons with aphasia. The authors found that severity of physical functioning was rated as more important to the persons with aphasia than was communication functioning. Furthermore, the ratings from significant others and SLPs were significantly correlated with each other but not with those of the PWAs. The message continues to be that proxies and PWAs do not necessarily agree on the importance of health-related quality of life domains, thereby emphasising the importance of initiating and continuing these topics of communication with PWAs themselves.

The comments from PWAs in the current study indicate substantial self-awareness about their speech. Just over a third mentioned some specific attributes that characterise their speech production and just under a third mentioned improvement over time. These comments about the need to speak more slowly or speech being better earlier in the day, for example, suggest self-awareness and self-regulation, curiosity about their own symptoms, and creativity, also thought to be positive strengths that affect wellbeing. A smaller number of participants mentioned specific techniques being employed for therapeutic purposes. Taken together, these themes bear striking similarity to metaphors used to described aphasia rehabilitation in a recent study by Ferguson et al. (2010). PWAs used the metaphoric concepts of *product*, *body*, *journey*, and *battle* most frequently; family members and SLPs used *journey* most frequently. The changes over time were a common theme for all parties involved in the experience of aphasia. The authors encourage the consideration of metaphor to compare and contrast perspectives between PWAs, their family members, and SLPs for purposes of treatment and counselling.

The fact that participants in this study responded positively concerning their speech would seem to bode well for the participants. For example, Seligman and Peterson (2003) note, "Psychologists have discovered that there are human strengths that act as buffers against mental illness: courage, future-mindedness, optimism, the capacity for flow, and insight to name several" (p. 314). There is reason to believe that these same strengths play a role in recovery from a number of diseases and disorders as well (Fitzgerald, Tennen, Affleck, & Pransky, 1993; Pressman & Cohen, 2005), and stroke and aphasia should be no exception. Using meta-analytic techniques, Rasmussen et al. (2009) demonstrated that optimism is a significant predictor of physical health and that subjective measures, including self-reports, produced significantly higher effect sizes than did objective measures. Also interesting and relevant was the fact that the effect sizes were not significantly different for patient populations versus healthy populations, although they were larger in the studies using patient populations.

In a short report on coping in psychiatric-mental health illness, Edward and Warelow (2005) explain that both genetic factors and learned protective behaviours can contribute to a person's resilience when facing adversity. They stress that knowing about resilient behaviours may improve clinical practice and affect outcomes. Therapy that includes support and education, and specifically a focus on resilient behaviours can especially help in aphasia where communication skills are involved. Clinicians are being urged to help patients renegotiate their identities (Shadden, 2005). Allowing for identification and recognition of other factors of resilience such as humour, flexibility, intellectual competence, self-reliance, persistence, and hopefulness may help aphasic individuals strengthen their sense of self in the altered context of their post-stroke lives.

This study does not claim to provide in-depth analysis of the acknowledged deep-seated identity and adjustment issues facing people with aphasia, nor a detailed linguistic examination of evaluative language. However, it presents an interesting new approach to this issue, because the raw data from this study are now openly available over the web to the research community. To facilitate direct examinations, we have inserted our coding for each response into each transcript on the @G: Speech line where the prompt was given. Using this transparent and open data window we can join with other researchers in conducting further analyses of the detailed gestural and intonational features accompanying these verbal descriptions. Moreover, as we can add further data to this openly available source from a wider array of participants and use additional prompts, which could elicit more information about the details of physical and social adaptation to aphasia. It may also be possible eventually to include data collected from non-institutional contexts.

Although data collected in this interview format remain bound to the institutional context, it is important to remember that this is the context in which PWAs encounter therapy and treatment. To the degree that these attitudes can shape treatment outcomes, it is important to better understand how PWAs evaluate their own therapy and recovery. By making these data directly available through AphasiaBank, we can add further reliability and replicability to the investigation of these relations.

REFERENCES

Armstrong, E. (2001). Connecting lexical patterns of verb usage with discourse meanings in aphasia. *Aphasiology, 15*, 1029–1046.

Armstrong, E., & Ulatowska, H. K. (2007). Making stories: Evaluative language and the aphasia experience. *Aphasiology, 21*(6), 763–774.

Beeke, S., Wilkinson, R., & Maxim, J. (2009). Prosody as a compensatory strategy in the conversations of people with agrammatism. *Clinical Linguistics & Phonetics, 23*(2), 133–155.

Behrns, I., Wengelin, A., Broberg, M., & Hartelius, L. (2009). A comparison between written and spoken narratives in aphasia. *Clinical Linguistics & Phonetics, 23*(7), 507–528.

Berndt, R., Wayland, S., Rochon, E., Saffran, E., & Schwartz, M. (2000). *Quantitative production analysis: A training manual for the analysis of aphasic sentence production*. Hove, UK: Psychology Press.

Bloom, R., Borod, J., Obler, L., & Gerstman, L. (1993). Suppression and facilitation of pragmatic performance: Effects of emotional content on discourse following right and left brain damage. *Journal of speech and Hearing Research, 36*, 1227–1235.

Bloom, R., Borod, J., Obler, L., & Koff, E. (1990). A preliminary characterization of lexical emotional expression in right and left brain-damaged patients. *International Journal of Neuroscience, 55*, 71–80.

Borod, J., Pick, L., Andelman, F., Obler, L., Welkowitz, J., Rorie, K., et al. (2000). Verbal pragmatics following unilateral stroke: Emotional content and valence. *Neuropsychology, 14*(1), 112–124.

Bose, A., McHugh, T., Schollenberger, H., & Buchanan, L. (2009). Measuring quality of life in aphasia: Results from two scales. *Aphasiology, 23*(7–8), 797–808.

Button, G., & Casey, N. (1985). Topic nomination and topic pursuit. *Human Studies, 8*, 3–55.

Byng, S., & Duchan, J. (2005). Social model philosophies and principles: Their applications to therapies for aphasia. *Aphasiology, 19*, 906–922.

Camras, L. A., Holland, E. A., & Patterson, M. J. (1993). Facial expression. In M. Lewis & J. M. Haviland (Eds.), *Handbook of emotions* (pp. 199–208). New York, NY: The Guilford Press.

Chapey, R., Duchan, J., Elman, R., Garcia, L., Kagan, A., Lyon, J., et al. (2000). Life participation approach to aphasia. In R. Chapey (Ed.), *Language intervention strategies in aphasia and related neurogenic communication disorders* (4th ed., pp. 235–245). Baltimore, MD: Lippincott, Williams & Wilkins.

Cherney, L. R., Halper, A. S., Holland, A. L., & Cole, R. (2008). Computerized script training for aphasia: Preliminary results. *American Journal of Speech-Language Pathology, 17*, 19–34.

Code, C., & Hermann, M. (2003). The relevance of emotional and psychosocial factors in aphasia to rehabilitation. *Neuropsychological Rehabilitation, 13*, 109–132.

Cranfill, T. B., & Wright, H. H. (2010). Importance of health-related quality of life for persons with aphasia, their significant others, and SLPs: Who do we ask? *Aphasiology, 24*, 957–968.

Cruice, M., Worrall, L., Hickson, L., & Murison, R. (2003). Finding a focus for quality of life with aphasia. Social and emotional health, and psychological well-being. *Aphasiology, 17*(4), 333–353.

Cruice, M., Worrall, L., Hickson, L., & Murison, R. (2009). Measuring quality of life: Comparing family members' and friends' ratings with those of their aphasic partners. *Aphasiology, 19*, 111–129.

Edward, K., & Warelow, P. (2005). Resilience: When coping is emotionally intelligent. *Journal of the American Psychiatric Nurses Association, 11*, 101–102.

Elman, R. (2005). Social and life participation approaches to aphasia intervention. In L. LaPointe (Ed.), *Aphasia and related neurogenic language disorders* (3rd ed., pp. 39–50). New York, NY: Thieme Medical Publishers.

Ferguson, A., Worrall, L., Davidson, B., Hersh, D., & Sherratt, S. (2010). Describing the experience of aphasia rehabilitation through metaphor. *Aphasiology, 24*(6–8), 685–696.

Fitzgerald, T., Tennen, H., Affleck, G., & Pransky, G. (1993). The relative importance of dispositional optimism and control appraisals in quality of life after coronary bypass surgery. *Journal of Behavioral Medicine, 16*, 25–43.

Fromm, D., Holland, A. L., & Swindell, C. S. (1984). Depression following left hemisphere stroke [abstract]. *Clinical Aphasiology Conference Proceedings*. Minneapolis, MN: BRK Publishers.

Hagstrom, F. (2004). Including identity in clinical practices. *Topics in Language Disorders, 24*(3), 225–238.

Heritage, J., & Clayman, S. (2010) *Talk in action: Interactions, identities, and institutions*. New York, NY: Wiley.

Hilari, K., & Byng, S. (2009). Health-related quality of life in people with severe aphasia. *International Journal of Language and Communication Disorders, 44*(2), 193–205.

Hilari, K., Northcott, S., Roy, P., Marshall, J., Wiggins, R., & Chataway, J. (2010). Psychological distress after stroke and aphasia: The first six months. *Clinical Rehabilitation, 24*, 181–190.

Hilari, K., Wiggins, R. D., Roy, P., Byng, S., & Smith, S. C. (2003). Predictors of health-related quality of life (HRQL) in people with chronic aphasia. *Aphasiology, 17*, 365–381.

Hinckley, J. (2006). Finding messages in bottles: Successful living with aphasia as revealed by personal narrative. *Topics in Stroke Rehabilitation, 13*, 63–67.

Holland, A. (2007). *Counseling in communication disorders: A wellness perspective*. San Diego, CA: Plural Publishing.

Holland, A. (2010). Lessons from a clinical life. *Topics in Stroke Rehabilitation, 17*, 13–19.

Holland, A., Halper, A., & Cherney, L. (2010). Tell me your story: Analysis of script topics selected by persons with aphasia. *American Journal of Speech-Language Pathology, 19*, 198–203.

Hunston, S., & Thompson, G. (Eds.) (2003). *Evaluation in text: Authorial stance and the construction of discourse*. Oxford, UK: Oxford University Press.

Kertesz, A. (2007). *Western Aphasia Battery Revised*. San Antonio, TX: PsychCorp.

MacWhinney, B. (2000). *The CHILDES Project: Tools for analysing talk, 3rd edition*. Mahwah, NJ: Lawrence Erlbaum.

Martin, J. R., & White, P. R. R. (2005). *The language of evaluation: Appraisal in English*. Basingstoke, UK: Palgrave Macmillan.

Oelschlaeger, M. L., & Thorne, J. C. (1999). Application of the correct information unit analysis to the naturally occurring conversation of a person with aphasia. *Journal of Speech, Language, and Hearing Research, 42*, 636–648.

Olness, G., Matteson, S. E., & Stewart, C. T. (2010). "Let me tell you the point": How speakers assign prominence to information in narratives. *Aphasiology, 24*(6–8), 697–708.

Pittam, J., & Scherer, K. R. (1993). Vocal expression and communication of emotion. In M. Lewis & J. M. Haviland (Eds.), *Handbook of emotions* (pp. 185–197). New York, NY: The Guilford Press.

Pomerantz, A. M. (1984). Agreeing and disagreeing with assessment: Some features of preferred/dispreferred turn shapes. In J. M. Atkinson & J. Heritage (Eds.), *Structure of social action: Studies in conversation analysis*. Cambridge, UK: Cambridge University Press.

Pound, C., Parr, S., Lindsay, J., & Woolf, C. (2000). *Beyond aphasia: Therapies for living with communication disability*. Bicester, UK: Speechmark.

Pressman, S., & Cohen, S. (2005). Does positive affect influence health? *Psychological Bulletin, 131*(6), 925–971.

Rasmussen, H. N., Scheier, M. F., & Greenhouse, J. B. (2009). Optimism and physical health: A meta-analytic review. *Annals of Behavioral Medicine, 37*, 239–256.

Riis, J., Lowenstein, G., Baron, J., Jepson, C., Fagerlin, A., & Ubel, P. A. (2005). Ignorance of hedonic adaptation to hemodialysis: A study using ecological momentary assessment. *Journal of Experimental Psychology: General, 134*, 3–9.

Robinson, J. (2006). Soliciting patients' presenting concerns. In J. Heritage & D. Maynard (Eds.), *Communication in medical care. Interaction between primary care physicians and patients. Studies in Interactional Sociolinguistics (20)* (pp. 22–47). Cambridge, UK: Cambridge University Press.

Robinson, R. G., & Benson, D. F. (1981). Depression in aphasic patients: Frequency, severity, and clinical-pathological correlations. *Brain and Language, 14*, 282–291.

Seligman, M., & Peterson, C. (2003). Positive clinical psychology. In L. Aspinwall & U. Staudinger (Eds.), *Fundamental questions and future directions for a positive psychology*. Washington DC: American Psychological Association.

Shadden, B., Hagstrom, F., & Koski, P. R. (2008). *Neurogenic communication disorders: Life stories and the narrative self*. San Diego, CA: Plural Publishing.
Shadden, B. B. (2005). Aphasia as identity theft. *Aphasiology*, *19*, 211–224.
Shadden, B. B., & Hagstrom, F. (2007). The role of narrative in the life participation approach to aphasia. *Topics in Language Disorders*, *27*(4), 324–338.
Simmons-Mackie, N., & Damico, J. (2009). Engagement in group therapy for aphasia. *Seminars in Speech & Language*, *30*, 18–26.
Simmons-Mackie, N., & Damico, J. (2010). Exploring clinical interaction in speech-language therapy: Narrative, discourse and relationships. In R. Fourie (Ed.), *Therapeutic processes for communication disorders: A guide for clinicians and students*. Hove, UK: Psychology Press.
Simmons-Mackie, N., Kagan, A., Christie, D., Huiuibregtas, M., McEwan, S., & Williams, J. (2007). Communicative access and decision making for people with aphasia: Implementing sustainable health-care systems change. *Aphasiology*, *21*(1), 39–66.
Tukey, J. W. (1977). *Exploratory data analysis*. Reading, MA: Addison-Wesley.
Ulatowska, H., & Olness, G. (2003). On the nature of direct speech in narratives of African Americans with aphasia. *Brain and Language*, *87*, 69–70.
Ulatowska, H., Olness, G., Keebler, M., & Tillery, J. (2006). Evaluation in stroke narratives: A study in aphasia. *Brain & Language*, *99*(1–2), 61–62.
Ulatowska, H. K., & Olness, G. (2001). Dialectal variants of verbs in narratives of African Americans with aphasia: Some methodological considerations. In M. Paradis (Ed.), *Manifestations of aphasia symptoms in different languages* (pp. 9–26). Amsterdam, The Netherlands: Pergamon.
Youmans, G., Holland, A., Munoz, M., & Bourgeois, M. (2005). Script training and automaticity in two individuals with aphasia. *Aphasiology*, *19*, 435–450.
Youmans, G., Youmans, S., & Hancock, A. (2011). Script training treatment for adults with apraxia of speech. *American Journal of Speech Language Pathology* , *20*(1), 23–37.

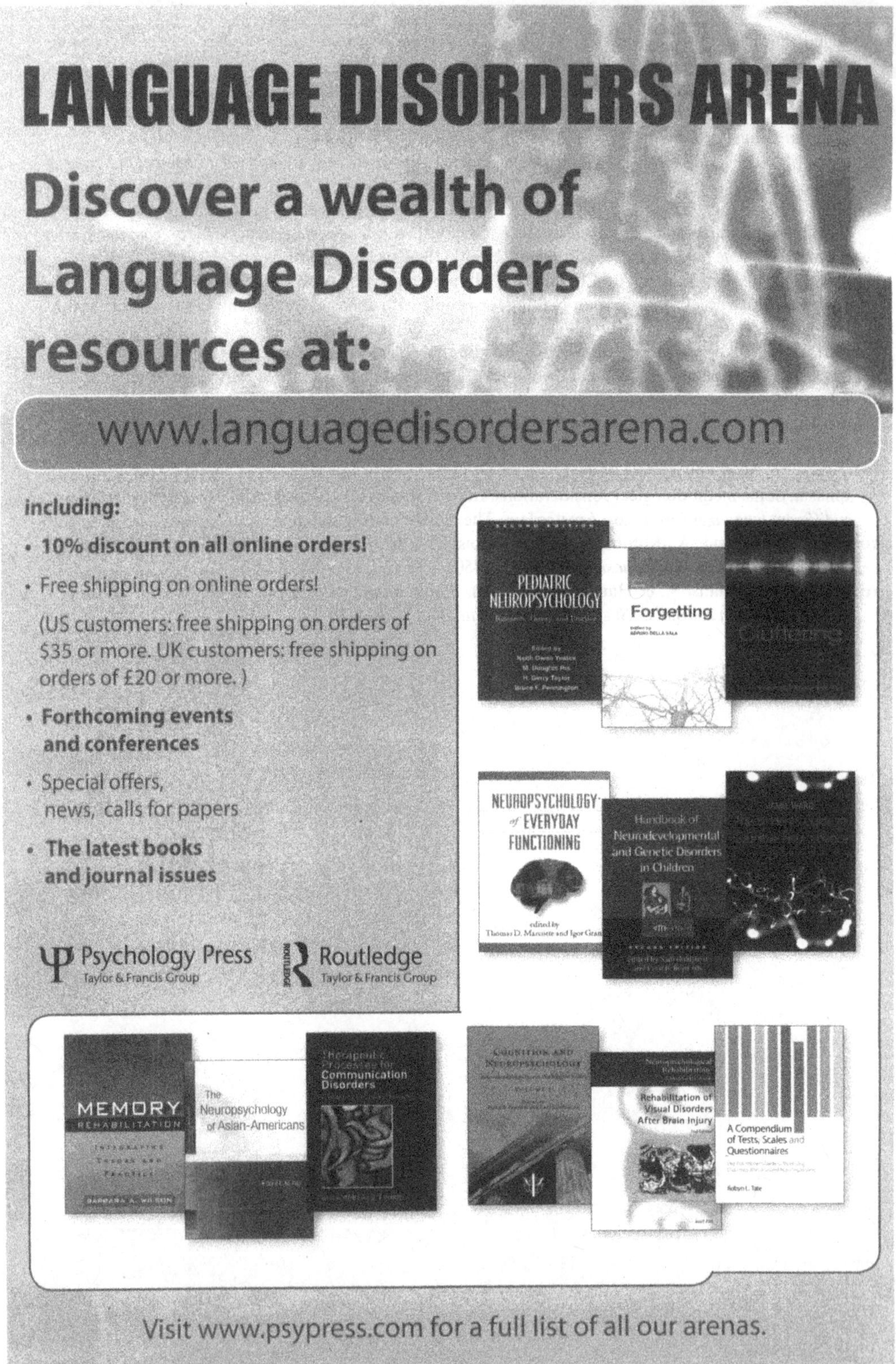
LANGUAGE DISORDERS ARENA
Discover a wealth of Language Disorders resources at:
www.languagedisordersarena.com
including:
• 10% discount on all online orders!
• Free shipping on online orders!
(US customers: free shipping on orders of $35 or more. UK customers: free shipping on orders of £20 or more.)
• Forthcoming events and conferences
• Special offers, news, calls for papers
• The latest books and journal issues
Psychology Press
Taylor & Francis Group
Routledge
Taylor & Francis Group
PEDIATRIC NEUROPSYCHOLOGY
Forgetting
NEUROPSYCHOLOGY of EVERYDAY FUNCTIONING
edited by Thomas D. Marcotte and Igor Grant
Handbook of Neurodevelopmental and Genetic Disorders in Children
MEMORY REHABILITATION
The Neuropsychology of Asian-Americans
Therapeutic Processes for Communication Disorders
COGNITION AND NEUROPSYCHOLOGY
Rehabilitation of Visual Disorders After Brain Injury
A Compendium of Tests, Scales and Questionnaires
Visit www.psypress.com for a full list of all our arenas.

APHASIOLOGY

APHASIOLOGY is covered by the following abstracting and indexing services: *BLLDB (Bibliography of Linguistic Literature), CINAHL, Current Contents, Elsevier Science BV, EMBASE/Excerpta Medica, Linguistic Abstracts, Linguistic and Language Behavior Abstracts, Medical Documentation Service, PsycINFO, PsycBITE, Research Alert, Science Citation Index, SciSearch, SCOPUS, UnCover.*

Submitting a paper to APHASIOLOGY

Aphasiology is concerned with all aspects of language impairment and related disorders resulting from brain damage. Submissions are encouraged on theoretical, empirical and clinical topics from any disciplinary perspective, and submissions which involve cross disciplinary study are particularly welcome. *Aphasiology* will publish experimental and clinical research papers, reviews, theoretical notes, comments and critiques. Research reports can be group studies, single-case studies or surveys, on psychological, linguistic, medical and social aspects of aphasia. Submissions and ideas for the Review Articles and the Forum are welcome, and interdisciplinary peer commentary is encouraged. *Aphasiology* articles have a maximum limit of 7,500 words. This 7,500 is to include main text and references only. It excludes title, author's contact details, abstract, figures, tables, captions, and footnotes.

Submissions and books for, or offers to, review should be sent to an Editor, address on inside front cover.

Structured Abstracts

Authors submitting papers should note that the journal uses Structured Abstracts. There is good evidence that Structured Abstracts are clearer for readers and facilitate better appropriate indexing and citation of papers.

The essential features of the Structured Abstract are given below. Note in particular that any clinical implications should be clearly stated.

Abstract (between 150–400 words)

Background: Describe the background to the study.

Aims: State the aims and objectives of the study including any clear research questions or hypotheses.

Methods & Procedures: To include: outline of the methodology and design of experiments; materials employed and subject/participant numbers with basic relevant demographic information; nature of the analyses performed.

Outcomes & Results: Outline the important and relevant results of the analyses.

Conclusions: State the basic conclusions and implications of the study. State, clearly and usefully, if there are implications for management, treatment or service delivery.

Review Abstract

Background: Outline the background to the review.

Aims: State the primary objective of the paper, the reasons behind your critical review and analyses of the literature, and your approach and methods if relevant.

Main Contribution: Give the main outcomes of the paper and results of analyses; and any implications for future research and for management, treatment or service delivery.

Conclusions: State your main conclusions.

All submissions should be made online at *Aphasiology*'s Manuscript Central site (http://mc.manuscriptcentral.com/paph).

Papers are accepted for consideration on condition that you will accept and warrant the following conditions:

1. You will transfer copyright to Psychology Press, should the work be accepted for publication.
2. The work is your original work, and cannot be construed as plagiarising any other published work.
3. You own the copyright in the work.
4. You are empowered by your fellow author(s) to make a submission to this journal, and to make any agreement relating to the work.
5. Your work has not previously been published in the English language.
6. Your work is not under consideration for publication elsewhere, in any form.
7. You have secured the necessary permission in writing from the appropriate authorities for the reproduction in your work of any text, illustration, or other material which is reproduced or derived from a copyrighted source.
8. You have agreed with your fellow author(s) the order of names for publication of the work.
9. You warrant that the work does not include content that is abusive, defamatory, libellous, obscene, fraudulent, or in violation of applicable laws.

If it is found acceptable for publication, you shall retain the right to use the substance of the above work in future works, on condition that you acknowledge its prior publication in the journal, and the publishers Psychology Press.

Free article access

As corresponding author, you will receive free access to your article on Taylor & Francis Online. You will be given access to the *My authored works* section of Taylor & Francis Online, which shows you all your published articles. You can easily view, read, and download your published articles from there. In addition, if someone has cited your article, you will be able to see this information. We are committed to promoting and increasing the visibility of your article and have provided this guidance <http://journalauthors.tandf.co.uk/beyondpublication/promotearticle.asp> on how you can help.

Reprints and journal copies

Corresponding authors can receive a complimentary copy of the issue containing their article. Reprints can be purchased through Rightslink® when proofs are received. If you have any queries about reprints, please contact the Taylor & Francis Author Services team at reprints@tandf.co.uk. To order extra copies of the issue containing your article, please contact our Customer Services team at adhoc@tandf.co.uk.

Style Guides

Please refer to the following website for the journal style guide, and for more information on our other journals and books: http://www.psypress.com

This publication has been produced with acid-free paper manufactured to strict environmental standards and with pulp derived from sustainable forests.